The Grey Drinking Reset:

a 30 Day Journey to Wellness

D1665775

by Carrie Schell

The Gray Drinking Reset

Carrie Schell

Costa Rica

Carrie.Schell@gmail.com

Ordering Information:

Special discounts are available on quantity purchases by corporations, associations, educational institutions, and others. For details, contact Carrie Schell above.

Printed in the United States of America

First Edition

Softcover ISBN 978-1-5136-9414-6

eBook ISBN 978-1-5136-9392-7

Publisher

Winsome Entertainment Group LLC

Foreword

One day, a drink is a simple way of relaxing, or part of lunch with friends, or a party staple. But, before you know it, drinking has become a problem. That pretty much sums up my own experience with gray drinking.

My own drinking started with happy hour every Friday to blow off steam after a stressful week at work. It was fun and social, and felt normal. And it alleviated the pressure that had built up all week.

From there, I entered the insanely high-pressure world of advertising. We wined and dined clients *every* night. Without really realizing it, I had shifted from having drinks with friends one night a week to nearly every day imbibing one or two drinks – not just wine, but serious alcohol.

But it didn't stop there. When I was at home, I would find myself opening a bottle of wine and having a glass with dinner. One day, I woke up and realized that it had become an entire bottle of wine with, and sometimes for, dinner.

My partying escalated to drinking during every outing. Friday and Saturday night with friends, Sunday brunch, and all the rest of Sunday too. I couldn't imagine a day without alcohol. I tried to cut back here and there, but ultimately a stressful day would happen and I would be right back in the bottle.

The thing I came to realize was that it was about me. I hated my job. I couldn't sustain a relationship. I simply wasn't happy. Drinking had become a way to escape from the reality of my unhappiness. After a really brutal breakup, I decided it was time to quit. I just woke up one morning with a nasty hangover and decided, "I'm done."

Within three weeks, I dropped ten pounds. That was the biggest surprise. It made me realize how many empty calories I had been drinking every day.

Bigger than that, I was feeling angry. I found out later that this is a normal reaction. I was now feeling all the feelings that I had been suppressing by drinking. I had a choice: I could go back to suppressing or I could do the hard work of feeling those feelings and beginning to heal and grow.

It was deeply awful and completely wonderful all at the same time.

Within seven months I had a new career that I loved. I exercised regularly and ate better, which made me feel better. I met my future husband and got married. I realized that the alcohol in my life had stunted my growth.

Now I was ready to fly.

When Carrie first brought me the idea of this book, I was all in. Several entrepreneurs had brought me the idea of a gray drinking book, but no one stepped up like Carrie did. She said, "I see a problem in the world, and I want to use my expertise to help."

We dipped our toes in the water with a 10-Day Reset and two weeks later, Carrie had written a comprehensive book that became the basis for this book. She stepped up to deliver like no one else had in this arena. She saw a problem, committed to do whatever it took to solve the problem and help others, and then did the work to produce a phenomenal book.

If you even suspect that you might be a gray drinker, I hope you will embrace Carrie's story and guidance as the invitation to heal your mind, body, and spirit. This book is a great beginning for those who have lost their way, or who haven't realized what awaits them in a sober, empowered world.

Carrie's raw honesty about her own journey will inspire you through all the ups and downs, and at the end, you might just be amazed at your results. I wish I had had her in my corner back when I was dealing with ending my own addiction.

~Juliet Clark

My Personal Journey

Over the years, I have had many times when I thought that I was drinking too much or that I should really take a break from drinking. I tried several times to stop drinking. I have even gone for a couple weeks or months without drinking (although, even during those times of "not drinking," I would sneak in a glass of wine here and there and feel super proud of myself that I had such restraint).

But sure enough, while on my self-imposed drinking hiatus, I'd think,"*Why am I being so restrictive? I don't need to be so all-or-nothing about alcohol. I can have a glass of wine with dinner.*" Or I'd rationalize my drinking with, "*In Europe they have a glass of wine with lunch and dinner. If I were in Europe I wouldn't even be second guessing how much wine I drink. Our views on alcohol are so uptight in North American.*"

So I'd start drinking again.

I'd soon be right back where I left off—drinking and continuing to drink because that first glass of wine went down so quickly, and I'd soon be onto my second. I would feel good about those evenings when I stopped at two glasses. I'd tell myself at the beginning of the evening, or at an event, or whatever, "*I'm only going to have one glass of wine,*" but I'd easily and frequently finish the whole bottle. I even stopped drinking red wine because years ago, when my husband and I were going through a challenging time in our marriage, he blurted out, "You get mean when you drink red wine." So I promptly stopped drinking red wine. Done, just like that. But all I did was switch to white wine which I had previously hated. Problem solved, but not really.

I have never hit a rock bottom. In fact, I wonder if we grey drinkers fall into the type A personality realm, juggling many balls, keeping everything super organized, in order, and finding relief, relaxation, or reward with a few drinks in the evening. We keep it all together. We have our jobs, our families, our friendships. We can cut back, kinda. We can stop, well maybe next month or after that wedding or party we've been invited to. But it's always there. That quiet knowing that we have slipped into the grey area. We are grey drinkers.

Signs You May Be a Grey Drinker:

1. You silently worry, regret, and fret about your drinking.

2. You drink between two extremes, all or nothing.

3. You *can* stop drinking and you have stopped drinking for periods of time—even weeks or months—but it's hard to stay stopped.

4. Your drinking doesn't look problematic to those around you.

5. You ricochet between ignoring that still small voice inside of you telling you to stop drinking and deciding that you're overthinking, and you need to just "live a little."

Alcohol is your reward at the end of the day. It's how you have fun, relax, unwind, connect, have sex, and fall asleep at night. Everything in moderation, right? Yet, you've lost count how many times you've woken up the day after "living a little" and said, *"Never again. I can't keep drinking like this."*

When I made the decision to stop for good, I knew I was done forever. I knew I was done because I had so many stops and starts, and this time, I knew not to dwell in the grey. The grey had become black and white. I told myself that, no matter what happened in the future, good or bad, there would be no more silent debates, bargaining, justifying, or wondering if I could have just "one," because one always turned into more.

I was ready for a full stop. It was scary to stop. Alcohol is our best frenemy, there to celebrate the good times and to comfort us in the low times. It is always there, ready, dependable, and will never say no. What about our friends, dinners out, social occasions, how do I fit in and function without alcohol? These are the thoughts that ran through my head.

Here's the thing: if you are reading this, you are already stronger than you know. It takes courage and self-awareness to even explore this.

The 30-Day Reset

Let's take this 30-day journey together. Commit to thirty days. I know, thirty days seems like an eternity when you are already making a mental note to check to see if you have wine chilling for tonight. But you can do it. You've got this.

If you are curious to explore your grey drinking, this is the perfect time to honour yourself by entering this 30-day reset.

Together, we will explore what comes up for us along with the milestones and victories to celebrate. Most importantly, we give ourselves the time and space to explore our true selves, without alcohol. The best version of us.

What to Expect from the Process

I thought it may help if I outline what our work is going to look like while on our journey together.

Each day, you will be guided through a number of activities to support your wellbeing. It's going to be the same each day, so hopefully you will slide into a comfortable routine. The program is straightforward. All you need is a journal and a willingness to join me.

What will you be doing? It's very simple.

5 Minutes: You'll spend five minutes of quiet, reflective time to begin your day. Seems boring and you may be asking, "What's the point?" But I assure you, it will become an important part of your day. I promise.

Thirty Minutes: At some point during the day, you're going to need to get moving. It can be anything: your favourite workout, your least favourite workout, a walk, yoga, whatever. It doesn't matter, just get moving. To cool down, it's best to slow it down and meditate. Feel free to enjoy the daily guided meditation, just follow the link. Oh, and drink eight glasses of water a day to help to cleanse the system.

Journaling: Each day there will be a journaling prompt followed by an excerpt from my own journal which are in italics. I just want you to know that I am with you on this. Please take the time to write in your journal any and all that you are experiencing and feeling through our time together. Hopefully this will help us connect.

I've included excerpts from my journal for you because I wanted to share with you some of the thoughts and emotions I experienced during my own reset. My intention is to show you anything and everything you experience on this journey is *normal*.

Writing these things down validates what we are feeling and living out and gives us a sense of ownership of our journey. It is in truly owning where we're at that we have the potential to change and *choose* our next steps.

The remaining three sections include Today's Thought, a Word for Today, an Affirmation, and an Exercise. The exercise gives you a prompt to reflect and write on. Pretty straightforward, right? Make sense? And that's it. Let's get to it.

Day 1

You've bought the book, you're ready to begin… now what?

This is our "soft" launch. Before we truly begin our work together, we need to make sure we get a few things in order. Sound good? Today is all about preparing for the Reset, mentally and physically.

First off, if you're like me, it's far easier to begin a program when I've cleared out my cupboards of whatever it is that may tempt me. Out of sight, kinda out of mind, right?

What I would like you to do is clear out all the alcohol from your home. It will be much easier to not drink when you don't have alcohol around. Make sense?

What do you do if your partner isn't going to do the Reset with you? To be honest, that can make it a little trickier. If there is something your partner drinks that you don't enjoy, perfect. Reduces temptation. This is all about positioning yourself for success for 30 days.

If your partner drinks beer and you *love* beer, it's like putting a kid in a candy shop. Hopefully your partner will value and respect the journey you are on and agree to either stop drinking with you, limit their consumption, or agree not to drink at home. The key is communication. Express your needs and find a workable solution.

This conversation will be an eye opener, whichever direction it takes. If your partner is agreeable, happy to change their patterns to ensure you are successful, you're all set! If, on the other hand, your partner is not willing to budge or change patterns of drinking, you are going to need to do some serious reflection on the role alcohol is playing in your relationship. What is the value you each place on alcohol? How so you prioritize alcohol in terms of your relationship? We'll get into this later, but for now, food for thought.

Alcohol is cleared out, check! Next, make sure you have a journal or notebook to do the work I am going to ask you to do on the daily.

Find a place that you can devote to quiet reflection in the mornings and your daily guided meditation. You may want to set up candles, a comfy cushion, whatever gives you a sense that this is a special place for you to do important work.

Give some thought to what sort of daily physical activity you're going to be doing. You'll be doing 30 minutes daily. If you're going to go on daily walks, do you have good shoes? Yoga, do you have a mat? Joining a class, are you all signed up and good to go? Today is the day to get this all sorted, because tomorrow we begin.

Lastly, take a moment to take in the fact that you are here, reading this. The fact that you had the courage to question your relationship with alcohol and begin this program demonstrates you are stronger than you know and want to step into the best version of you.

I am so proud of you. We are on this journey together. There will be tough days and there will be days when everything seems lighter, more wonderful! Through our work together, those brighter days will begin to outnumber the challenging ones, I promise.

So, get a good night's sleep and let's begin fresh, tomorrow.

Sending light and love,

Carrie

PS: Please do the Bliss Test *before* you begin the Reset!

The Bliss Test

Take this test before you begin your 30 day program and again after you complete it. This test is not meant to be used as a scientific tool, but a fun way to give you an overall idea of the extent of the stress and bliss in your life.

Rate each item on a scale of 0 to 10 in terms of how accurately it describes you.

A 0 would be "Does not describe me at all."

A 5 would be "Sometimes describes me."

A 10 would be "Always describes me."

1. I am a happy person.

2. I have a clear purpose in my life that I'm pleased about.

3. I am achieving what I want in my life.

4. The stress in my life is moderate to manageable.

5. I am patient and calm in times of struggle.

6. I take good care of my physical and emotional health.

7. My life is exciting and challenging.

8. I get pleasure regularly from helping others.

9. There are people in my life who love me and who I enjoy spending time with.

10. My work is meaningful to me and serves others.

Total score out of a possible 100 ____

Results

If you scored 0-30, you don't have a lot of bliss in your life, and you're probably experiencing one or more symptoms of stress.

If you scored 31-60, you could probably use more bliss in your life, but you may not notice you feel all that stressed out.

If you scored 61-100, spread the love.

Week 1

Befriending Your Boday

On this wellness journey, allow yourself to get settled into a bit of a routine. Begin each day with some quiet reflection. Each week will have a different focus to guide you through this.

Also, get physically active for at least thirty minutes every day, if you're not already. It can be whatever you like: a walk, yoga, Spin class, Pilates, a hike, swimming. Whatever gets you moving. From the time we were in our momma's womb, we were moving – we were born to move. It is key to mind, body, and spirit wellness.

You're also going to need to make time for journaling. Each week there will be a theme. This week's theme **befriending**, for example, is exploring your relationship with food. I'll give you cues on what to explore in your writing and you can take it from there.

For now, get yourself a dedicated journal that you will use throughout this 30-Day Reset. It can be as simple and inexpensive as a spiral notebook. The point is that this journal is for your eyes only and for this process only.

There is no right or wrong in this process, so just let it flow. Some days you may find that you have volumes to jot down and the next day crickets. It's all good. Just put the time into it.

You'll notice that I have shared with you some of my own journaling while on this journey. Those are the sections in italics. My intention here is that you see the wide range of thoughts and emotions I experienced and to show you that you aren't alone on this crazy ride. There are highs and lows and many questions. It's normal. Just go with it. I hope my sharing brings you a bit of comfort with where you are at.

Then we get into the meaty work.

There will be *Today's Thought,* a Word of the Day, an affirmation (no, I'm not asking you to repeat this affirmation multiple times daily. This affirmation is intended to validate your journey and be a source of encouragement and strength.), and an exercise.

You will also be writing for the exercise. Remember, *you're worth the time* you are putting into this. You've come into an awareness that you are a grey drinker and that you want to create a healthy relationship with alcohol. That is going to require time and effort on your part.

You may be backsliding and saying, "I don't have time to do all of this in a day." Bullshit. We all have the time, it's simply a matter of what, with whom, and how we choose to prioritize our time.

For the next 30 days, **YOU** are the priority. Reschedule your day. Get up a little earlier or stop watching Netflix. DO whatever it takes to make that happen.

Let's go Team You.

Putting Intention into Action

For this and every other week of the program, as you begin to become more aware of yourself and how you are showing up in your life, you will have the opportunity to try out new ideas that come to you during your practice, particularly in the reflective exercises of journaling and meditation.

See if you can find ways to put your new awareness to work in your daily life. It may be as simple as deciding you want to smile more, share a kind word with a loved one, or give your child or partner a hug. Simple things such as these may not look like life changing acts, but if you repeat them daily and practice them with conscious awareness, they will go a long way in supporting you as you turn your stress into bliss.

Establish Your Routine

Here is your first week's schedule. I have marked the start of the program as Monday for simplicity, a fresh start. However, feel free to start on whatever day you like.

Theme

The theme for this first week is **befriending your body**.

Your body is a key player in your success with this challenge. It is through your body that you will learn the most and through your body that you will change everything in your life that needs to change.

This first week will guide you to reconnect with your physical self and explore how your body is currently feeling. It will be the foundation to developing a loving relationship with yourself and discovering your sense of self and self-worth.

Take a deep breath in and a long, slow breath out. Ready?

The first question you need to ask yourself is, "What kind of relationship do I have with my body?"

Before you jump with a negative response, take time to really investigate this. If you do have negative thoughts about your body, how did this happen? At what point in your life did you start being negative about you? At what point in your life did you give yourself permission to be out of shape and harm your body with lack of exercise and poor eating?

We all struggle with body issues. I can tell you that this is a strong barrier for me. I struggle to like my body and am working to accept and love how I look. **The key here is to not judge yourself, but instead choose to heal.** Making that powerful choice will give you the strength to see this through.

Over the next four weeks in our work together, and I emphasize together, we will learn from each other. Our goal is to feel better, to be in control, and set ourselves on the path to a healthier life, physically, emotionally, and spiritually.

PS: I started the challenge on a Monday, my famous day for fresh starts, but start on any day that works for you.

MONDAY

Before you get out of bed, before your feet hit the floor, simply say, "Thank you. I am blessed. I am grateful." Do this every morning when you wake.

You may simply be saying this and initially it may have little meaning or ring hollow. But give it time. Each day you practice this, these simple phrases will mean more and more to you.

You are here doing this challenge with a purpose. There is something within you that seeks something other than the way you're doing things up until now. Remember that. There is a spark within that is worthy of attention. Thank *you* for being here. I am blessed and full of gratitude to be part of your journey.

Five Minutes

Begin your day with sitting quietly for five minutes. Do not focus on your day and the tasks at hand. **Simply sit and breathe.**

Thirty Minutes

For a lot of grey drinkers, exercise, working out and staying fit isn't an issue. In fact, many grey drinkers have a drink or two as a reward for working out. "I'm not going to have that glass of wine until I go for a run…" Sound familiar?

Please, please don't stop this commitment to your physical well-being. What we can't do is use our physical wellbeing as a justification as to why we should have a drink. "I'm fit and not overweight, so I can have a couple of drinks at the end of a day." The challenge is trying to develop a sense of purpose and incentive to keep physically active that does not include the reward of alcohol.

After you have been physically active, I'd like you to listen to one of the guided meditations included with the challenge. Slow things down. Let go and simply be.

Drink eight glasses of water today. Water? Yuck. The water will help cleanse your system and flush your liver, removing toxins from your body. Do it, your body will love you.

Monday Meditation link:
https://www.youtube.com/watch?v=-LRvhHD82nI&t=7s&ab_channel=CarrieSchell

Today's Thought

If you don't accept yourself, you won't life fully,

and if you don't live fully,

you'll need to get full some other way.

Accepting who you are, body and soul, does not guarantee that you will be perfect. It does, however, put you in the ideal position for becoming truly happy and healthy – developing habits to last a lifetime. If you don't accept yourself, you won't live fully, and if you don't live fully, you'll need to get full some other way, and unfortunately, it's usually with things that don't support you... alcohol, drugs, food, shopping, porno, whatever fills the void.

Word for Today: DENIAL (Don't Even Notice I'm Lying)

"Denial is a defense mechanism. It protects us from the truth, especially when the truth is painful. We don't want to see reality because of what it ultimately means. It's hard to reconcile the truth of our grey drinking when so many of the people we know, love, and socialize with are also grey drinkers. Our self-esteem can't face the reality that our drinking has become a problem, so we alter our reality. We rationalize and explain away to ourselves that all is good because we can't accept the reality that our drinking has gone beyond healthy limits. Denial needs to be penetrated or shattered before we can truly admit that we are totally powerless over alcohol."

~Allen Berger, *12 Stupid Things That Mess Up Recovery*

Affirmation:

I am now willing to acknowledge the truth of my grey drinking.

Journaling

Record everything you eat for the next week. Why do this? By actually writing down what you eat, you draw your attention to what you are putting into your body. You are cultivating awareness of what you eat. You will also become aware of what you were drinking while you ate. Glass of wine with lunch? Beer after work? Drink before dinner? Nightcap?

Through awareness, you can begin to make conscious choices which will support a healthy you. So, no cheating here. It is important for you to get a handle on what you eat, when you eat, how much you are eating and even why you eat.

You may even notice that you start to replace alcohol with other things like sugar and caffeine. Be mindful and observant with what's going on with you. Things are going to start coming up for you during this challenge: cravings, fear, worry, doubt, happiness, gratitude. The whole gamut. You need to write it down. You need to release it and let it go. And most importantly, always write down one positive thing that you like about yourself and one positive thing about the day ahead of you.

Perform one small act to support your intention of befriending your body (put the chocolate bar down!) This can be something as simple as not criticizing yourself today or making an effort to smile more. Maybe you'll call a friend you've been thinking about. One small act of kindness that signals you are worthy.

Schedule something special for you Thursday night – a walk, a bubble bath, a yummy dinner, or a movie out.

Excerpt:

Well, I knew day one would be rough. I kept preparing myself throughout the week, praying, asking the Holy Spirit to give me strength. Knowing that living here, in Costa Rica, in a beach community where we gather every sunset, cocktail in hand, it would be rough. And it was. So rough that I started the day after I had planned, justifying the change to be in keeping with the first day of Lent. Not true. I just wasn't ready.

Three days later, full day, yard work in the hot sun, getting a lot accomplished for our renters who arrive in 3 days' time. Sunset, craving a margarita. Making dinner, missing my glass of white wine. A glass of ice water with lime in a stemless glass to simulate the experience. Only to have it all fall apart with my losing it on my son and husband. Walking out, missing dinner. Returning, calmer, trying to still the waters. Damage done, again. Mother's guilt never ends, always present, always could do more, should do more. Be better, be stronger, be everything to everyone. Big shoulders sometimes slump.

Exercise:

Reveal to yourself how often you have rationalized your drinking, both to yourself and others, in order to continue your patterns of drinking.

Remember that this is for your eyes only. ***It is of vital importance that you are on this journey with honesty.***

TUESDAY

Five Minutes

Begin your day with sitting quietly for five minutes. Do not focus on your day and the tasks at hand. Simply sit and breathe.

Thirty Minutes

- Physical activity.

- Drink 8 glasses of water today.

- Remember, your body will love it.

- Enjoy a guided meditation: https://www.youtube.com/watch?v=S03R-Gxrszg&t=328s&ab_channel=CarrieSchell

Today's Thought:

You cannot drink and still be yourself.

Why all the food talk when this is a grey drinking challenge? Believe it or not, there is a connection between what you eat and how you feel about yourself. The more you become aware of your worthiness, of how great you are, the more likely you are to begin to eat healthily. They go hand in hand.

That's why we're spending some time developing a positive attitude toward food and eating. You can adopt better habits only if they honour who you are. There is a healthy way of eating that is natural and realistic for you. The point is to know and respect yourself so you can make appropriate choices based on who you are and how you live.

When you make the choices that will nurture change for your body and your life, they must be ones that work for you and that honour who you are. It may take some adjustments, and there may be some painful bumps along the way, but you are worth the effort.

The point is to have a healthier lifestyle, not to live a life full of resentments due to newly adopted changes. Eating is also a very social thing, a social thing that provides the perfect opportunity to drink. We need to learn how to enjoy eating while letting go of drinking. It's tough, real tough. I love to have wine when I go out to eat, so do many of my friends. And yes, they ask why I'm not drinking when I don't have a "problem" with alcohol. But I know my internal struggles with alcohol. I know that I don't want to drink as much as I have been and so I'm willing to trust and work with the challenge.

Let's do this together. We've got this.

Ask yourself:

- What does reasonable eating look like to me?

- How much do I enjoy my food when I am not drinking?

- In looking at my present lifestyle, what challenges may arise from my not drinking?

- Will my spouse or family be a help or hindrance to my making these changes?

- What things do I need to consider on the road to healthy living?

As you are painfully aware, the alcohol we have put into our bodies has an incredible impact on all aspects of our lives. The same is true with food. We need to develop a healthy relationship with our food that does not involve alcohol. This is why it is import to be mindful of what we eat, and how we approach our rituals of eating and begin to cultivate a positive mindset.

Word for Today: *FEAR (False Experiences Appearing Real)*

"The dark giants of fear and ignorance are closely allied. For instance, it's within no one's power to slay fear, because fear exists only as a shadow of the unknown and shadows can't be slain. But, it is within our power to challenge and conquer what is unknown since noting can prevent us from learning."

~Guy Finley, *The Secret of Letting Go*

Affirmation:

I am now willing to be courageous.

Journaling

Record everything you eat for the next week. No cheating here. This is important for you to get a handle on what you eat, when you eat, how much you are eating and perhaps why you eat.

Take this time to be real with what you are feeling.

- Are you feeling supported in the challenge?

- Have you told people you are doing the challenge?

- Are you able to be honest with yourself with where you're at in your relationship with alcohol?

- Write down one positive thing that you like about yourself and one positive thing about the day ahead of you.

- Perform one small act to support your intention of befriending your body (finding the time to work out).

Excerpt:

So, will I never be able to drink again? I mean, I know that alcoholics believe that you can ever drink again, but I'm not an alcoholic, so where does that leave me? I drink too much, yes. I want to cut back, of course. But do I never want to drink again? Never, ever? What's the verdict out there on grey drinking and the ability to be able to have one or two in the future?

Exercise:

Reveal to yourself the underlying fears of letting go of your drinking.

For example: Are you frightened of the withdrawals? Maybe of your real feelings without the buffer of a substance? Or perhaps you fear losing the courage you feel alcohol gives you?

WEDNESDAY

Five Minutes

Begin your day with sitting quietly for five minutes. Do not focus on your day and tasks at hand, simply sit and breathe.

Thirty Minutes

- Physical activity.

- Drink 8 glasses of water today.

- Remember, your body will love it.

- Enjoy today's guided meditation:
https://www.youtube.com/watch?v=OTzP3a_50T4&t=10s&ab_channel=CarrieSchell

Today's Thought:

Give up the notion of blowing it.

This one simple phrase unwittingly signals both defeat on our path to wellness and permission to continue in unhealthy behaviors all at once, really. It goes like this, "It's Friday. I was really good and didn't have a drink all week. But then I cheated and had a glass or two of wine with dinner Friday. I'll start fresh Monday. Since I'm starting Monday again fresh, I may as well drink all weekend."

Sound familiar? So you had a drink. The "blowing it" concept is bullshit. It's a mind game we play to give ourselves permission to drink. If you blow it, fine. But please, please don't think that means you should continue drinking until the next self-imposed start to alcohol-free living begins.

Start fresh NOW. Don't wait for Monday. Be kind to yourself and more importantly, be honest with yourself and acknowledge why you had that drink. It isn't simply because "I like it."

Another alternative to having that drink is to not blow it. Easier said than done, I know. But there are two ways you can do this. One is to keep your expectations realistic so you will reach them.

Back to our food analogy. Let's say you are aspiring to eat three reasonable meals today and get your exercise in. This is realistic. Setting your sights on running 10 kilometers daily and eating only skinless chicken and lettuce leaves for the next four weeks isn't.

An example I think we can all relate to is wanting to get in shape and lose weight. All of us have, at one time or another, looked in the mirror and decided that today is the day. "I'm going to watch what I eat and start working out."

Here's the thing. Those extra pounds didn't materialize in a day. They crept up, ever so sneakily over time, until one day you woke up and thought, "When the heck did *that* happen?" Just as the weight took its sweet time to jump onto my ass, it will take the same sweet time to leave.

The same is true of our drinking. We didn't wake up one day at this point. It is going to take time, patience, and understanding to gently and ever so firmly say good-bye to it.

So, be kind to yourself in these early days and do not place yourself in situations that will trigger your longing for a drink and set you up for failure. Out of sight, out of mind…slowly and gradually. Eventually you will get to a place where you are not thinking and craving continually. You will begin to have experiences that do not require alcohol to be enjoyable or of perceived value.

The other way to stop blowing it is to forget the whole concept itself. Let's say you slept-in and couldn't get your exercise in for today. Did you blow it ? No. Unless you decide to give yourself permission to only eat junk food and never exercise again, then you haven't "blown it." So you missed your workout or had that piece of cake. Give yourself a different response: "Yeah, I didn't work out," or, "sure, I ate the cake," but don't forget to tell yourself, "sometimes that will happen. Let it go." That single change of how you view yourself and your actions will empower you in making positive changes.

The key is to acknowledge the problem and get right back into your routine. Don't continue to overeat for the rest of the day or wait until Monday (the famous diet start date). You had a slip. Do not give yourself permission to derail completely. Commit to bettering yourself that moment. Tell yourself, "I had a slip up, but you know what? I love myself enough to move on, move forward and continue my wellness journey." Call a friend. Journal. Go to a meeting. Go to church. Go for a walk or a hike. Get out in nature. Do whatever you need to do to reconnect with your inner self that wants an alcohol-free life. Continue with the program that very moment. And most importantly, forgive yourself. Love yourself.

Word for Today: *ANXIETY*

"Start suspecting that those anxious thoughts and feelings you catch
trying to sell you an umbrella are not there to shelter you from some
approaching storm...but, that their sole purpose is to lure you into one."
~Guy Finley, *The Secret Way of Wonder*

Affirmation

I am now willing to have a quiet mind, an open heart, and relaxed body.

Journal

Continue to take the time to honour your experience, both the highs and the lows of the challenge.

I know, we are only on Day 3 but already things are coming up. The waking up and wondering if you really *need* to give up drinking for 30 days. The rationalizing that how much you drink isn't a problem.

You're feeling better already and *have things under control* now and can monitor your consumption. Or maybe you're *really* starting to feel better. Maybe you're noticing you're not fuzzy in the morning. Maybe you are feeling good about making it through days one and two. Write it all down, the good, the bad, and the ugly.

Excerpt:

This is so fucked up. I know I want this. I want to be that person who can do this. I am disciplined, hard-working, and know that this is going to be so good for me. Then why is it so hard? Why does it seem like an unsurmountable challenge? Why do I have a deep-seated fear that I'll fail? How is it that other people can do it?

Exercise

- Reveal to yourself how you have used alcohol to release or suppress anxious thoughts and feelings.

- Be honest with how alcohol abuse has impacted your health, physically, mentally, and emotionally.

- Perform one small act to support your intention of befriending your body (tell yourself "I want to be healthy" fifty times today).

- Check in: How are you plans coming along for doing something special (and healthy) for you tomorrow night? Give it some thought. Small acts of kindness toward yourself are so important.

THURSDAY

Five Minutes

Begin your day with sitting quietly for five minutes. Do not focus on your day and the tasks at hand, simply sit and breathe.

Thirty Minutes

- Physical activity.
- Drink 8 glasses of water today.
- Remember, your body will love it.
- Enjoy a guided meditation:

https://www.youtube.com/watch?v=deH14yUg5Q4&ab_channel=CarrieSchell

Today's Thought

As a rule, eat three meals a day.

The act of having to eat three times daily serves us on many levels. In order to eat three times daily we need to put thought and energy into what we are going to eat.

You're actually going to have to be mindful throughout your day about how you are going to nurture your body. You'll be mindfully caring for yourself three times daily, and that's huge. Not only will you be alcohol-free, but you'll be also filling your body with nutritious meals three times a day.

Eating three meals a day is both a discipline and a gift that reinforces the act of positive behaviours. We need to be able to continue cultivating positive behaviours that do not include alcohol during the highs and lows we encounter. Creating new routines without alcohol will help us navigate these waters and provide stability.

Word for Today: *SHAME*

"Shame is an isolating feeling. We keep it hidden. Yet the more we isolate, hiding it behind the masks that once served us, the bigger it grows and the lonelier we feel. The more shame we feel, the more fear we feel. The greater the shame, the greater the fear of being alone. It's a crazy cycle. We may even act out in anger or turn it inward in the form of depression. When we act out of fear and hurt others, we feel shame and begin the cycle all over again.

It is important not to re-shame ourselves in the process of our journey. The wounded child inside us doesn't need more injury. We need to start turning down the volume on those ghosts from the past and present. We need to be aware of any shaming from those who are currently in our lives, then take the hand of the wounded child inside us and lead her or him away. Above all, we need to begin to be aware when we are shaming ourselves."

~Jane Middleton-Moz, *Shame and Guilt*

Affirmation

I release the past and I am grateful for the lessons learned.

Journaling

I know that, when I am going out for the evening, I really look forward to having a drink with my dinner. I like having a drink before dinner and a glass or two of wine while I eat. It just feels good. It is relaxing, it seems to slow the evening down and enliven the conversation and it tastes oh so good. So, what now? What about my husband and friends? Can I still enjoy an evening out without alcohol?

I would like you to write down one positive thing that you like about yourself and one positive thing about the day ahead of you.

Excerpt

Here I am, giving up drinking when he needs to give it up too. I mean, he drinks way more than I do. He seems to actually need to stop. He looks forward to the end of the day when he can have a drink. Why isn't he giving it up? Ugh. I'm a horrible human for thinking that. We are all on our own journey and I cannot make him want to change. Maybe if he sees that life without alcohol is good, better, then he will want that for himself also...maybe. (Doubtful? Hopeful?)

Exercise

Explain why you are so tired of feeling guilty.

Perform one small act to support your intention of befriending your body (put a Post-It note on the fridge, "I want to be healthy. I am worth it to not eat junk.")

Enjoy the bubble bath.

FRIDAY

Five Minutes

Begin your day with sitting quietly for five minutes. Do not focus on your day and the tasks at hand, simply sit and breathe.

Thirty Minutes

- Physical activity.
- Drink 8 glasses of water today.
- Remember, your body will love it.
- Enjoy a guided meditation:

https://www.youtube.com/watch?v=FpLp7waxoNU&ab_channel=CarrieSchell

Today's Thought

Set your intention for the day.

Before you get out of bed each morning, set your intention for the day. I know it sounds cliché but give it a shot.

At first it is going to seem forced, and it will be. That doesn't matter. The act of setting a positive intention for your day, forced or not, will have a direct impact on you.

Your intention can be simple, but make sure it is positive. You will begin to experience that beginning your day with positive intentions will actually set you up to have a good day.

Remember, you create your thoughts and your thoughts create your reality. You have the power *and choice* to make your thoughts positive or negative. Your thoughts become your actions which in turn become your reality. This is a huge concept, and it can be both scary and liberating.

Keep your heart and mind focused on positivity and gratitude and you will be blown away with the changes you experience in life. Promise.

Word for Today: *ANGER*

Underneath your anger, your need to control, your need to blame, your impatience, and your intolerance of others' weaknesses is a great deal of pain. In fact, pain often causes you to become angry in the first place.

If you find that you are angry most of the time and that your anger seems to linger on too long, take a peek underneath to see if there is pain that you have been avoiding.

If you don't expose your pain, you will never have a chance to heal. Instead, it will fester and worsen, causing you to become more bitter, defensive, and angry, every day.

Affirmation

I choose peace.

Journaling

How did I get to the point where I am needing, *wanting,* to do this challenge?

How did I become a grey drinker?

I am a grey drinker. I am not an alcoholic. I can go a day or two without drinking. I am productive in my daily life. I am a loving mom, wife, friend, daughter and sister. And yet, I am a grey drinker? How? Why?

Excerpt

It is so interesting that when you take a break from drinking (is this a break or is this for good?) that you begin to notice how so many people are grey drinkers and don't have any sense of it. It's crazy how as a society we have come to rely on alcohol so much. It has soaked its way into all aspects of our lives, the joys, the sorrows, the mundane, all of it. If this amount of drinking is the new normal, I get why people think I am stupid for not drinking. "Everyone drinks this much." But that doesn't make it a good thing.

Exercise

Did you grow up in an angry family? If not, describe what makes you angry and how you express anger (for example, yelling, silent treatment, physical violence).

Perform one small act to support your intention of befriending your body (buy a great piece of fruit for a snack).

SATURDAY

Five Minutes

Begin your day with sitting quietly for five minutes. Do not focus on your day and the tasks at hand, simply sit and breathe.

Thirty Minutes

- Physical activity.

- Drink 8 glasses of water today.

- Remember, your body will love it.

- Enjoy a guided meditation:

https://www.youtube.com/watch?v=-HhSnob0DUw&ab_channel=CarrieSchell

Today's Thought

Alter your definition of success.

Success is not something you acquire down the road. It can be precisely where you are on the journey, right now, today.

Start to view success from a loving, more serving place. Success means that every day you pay attention to your inner life, respect your body, and treat yourself and others well.

Begin to recognize that success is found on the inside. Once you begin to shift your success and sense of worthiness from externals to your inner life and relationships, you will experience success in your everyday life.

Ask yourself:

- Have I been kind to me today?

- Is how I am spending my time a reflection of what I value?

- Have I expressed gratitude to those I love?

- Am I mindful to stay in the positive?

- Have I taken care of my physical wellbeing today?

- And this is the big one: am I acting from a source of fear or love?

Early on, feeling fear is normal. We live in a world that cultivates fears and struggles rather than encouraging one to believe in the higher power of love. Don't be afraid of being afraid. A bit of trepidation can even be a good thing – the way stage fright can lead to a better performance. But fear can only serve us if it propels us to move away from thinking and acting out of fear towards a place where we are living from a source of love.

Release your fears in your journal. Connect to your Higher Power through meditation, prayer, or spend some more time in nature.

The idea is to start living fully, and being a success in your own eyes, sooner rather than later. You're succeeding in every moment, day by day. Remember that. You are entering a bright new world where you will find more opportunities for fulfillment and joy.

Accept this as you are actively changing the state of your mind, body and spirit.

Word for Today: *COMMUNICATION*

Relationships are not optional. They are a necessity. As humans, we have an innate need to bond, and if you cannot bond with others, you will bond with other things to try to meet that need – substances, shopping, food, sex, gambling, social media, whatever.

This is why you have to reach out to others. Being able to communicate with others is essential to building meaningful relationships and creating bonds with others.

Affirmation

I want to have healthy relationships.

Journaling

Have you noticed that, during the shutdown, you started drinking more? Maybe that is when your drinking slipped into these murky grey waters.

Maybe you've been a grey drinker for a while and the shutdown drew you in deeper.

Maybe most of your friends began drinking more also, in those feelings of uncertainty, fear, anxiety, and isolation.

Maybe our threshold for what is *normal* to drink shifted?

Consider these questions in your journal.

Excerpt

I was talking to my brother, and it is amazing how many of us starting drinking daily, a lot daily. I was drinking three quarters of a bottle of wine, no problem. It's not that I was chugging it or getting drunk. It would be over the course of many hours, but still, by the time I went to bed, the bottle was almost empty. That's fucked, right? My poor liver. And what a waste of money.

Exercise

Do you think you are a good listener? Honestly rate yourself as to your level of communication skills. Is there room for improvement?

Perform one small act to support your intention of befriending your body (buy a great piece of fruit for a snack or take a walk).

SUNDAY

If you have already completed the previous six days this week, then this day is a free day to spend an hour doing something that you really love to do, but no, I don't mean having a leisurely brunch with mimosas.

If you haven't done the work than today is your lucky day. Go for it! You will be so thankful you invested the time and energy into YOU.

Enjoy a guided meditation, go for a walk, spend time with people you care about.

Start thinking about Sunday as your day, a day of rest. It may sound old school and antiquated but you need to be able to slow down, let go, and make a conscious decision to let Sunday be that day (or Saturday if that works better for you).

This means you are prioritizing your well-being. Once you set Sunday aside, make sure you schedule no meetings, no business, no laundry, no work. Do only things that bring you a sense of peace and support your well-being, mind, body, and spirit.

This can be very hard to do. Believe me, I find it very challenging to simply be, but I am learning to love it. Just like when I started doing yoga, I would skip the shavasana because I was only in it for the fitness aspect. Now shavasana is why I do yoga.

Here's the link for the Sunday meditation: https://www.youtube.com/watch?v=AGXHWm7rVoQ&ab_channel=CarrieSchell
Please accept this gift I am offering you.

Week 2

Congratulations! You have completed the first week of challenge and are about to begin the second. How did it go? What do you notice about yourself after week 1? Are you starting to be a little kinder to your body? Are you finding it easy or difficult to find the 40 minutes each day for this practice? Is there anything different you need to try this week to make it easier?

Remember, take it one day at a time. For today, simply make the firm commitment to be there for yourself for those 40 minutes tomorrow. And then tomorrow make the same commitment for the next day.

This week, the theme is **becoming more aware**. You might be wondering how and why you're going to do that. Or you might think that you already are aware.

The truth is that most of us, most of the time, live in a state of selective awareness. We are aware of the things that support life the way we have it set up, and we selectively hide from our awareness of the things that might rock the boat; we are afraid of the things that could cause change in our lives - if we were to be honest with ourselves.

Think of your life grey drinking. While in its hold, we don't truly allow ourselves to acknowledge the impact it has on our lives and our bodies. Yes, we know that it has a negative impact, but each time we give in and return to old patterns of behaviour, we quickly push those thoughts away. We do not want to be aware of the consequences the habit we rely on creates.

Another big area of our lives in which we often put our awareness aside is our relationships. Are we really conscious of what we are doing when we react to something our partner or family and friends might say, or do?

Awareness is the first step toward change. Without it, we usually remain static, without growth. Who's kidding who? Becoming aware is tough. Coming into an awareness necessitates action. If we aren't aware, there is no need to change.

Practicing awareness is not only about noticing the things you don't like. The beautiful thing is that awareness also allows us to experience all the great moments in each day and to have gratitude for them.

Practicing awareness demands that we slow our pace a little. If we are rushing from one thing to the next, we have little time to become aware of what is really happening in the moment.

For this week, we'll keep it simple. Try to focus your awareness on three areas: your body, your breath, and your thoughts.

Check in with your body periodically during the day. How does it feel in the moment? How are you holding it? Where does it feel good, and where does it not feel so good? How about your breath: Is it deep and full or shallow and rapid? And what are you thinking about? Check in with your mental process from time to time. Notice what seems to keep coming up during your day.

Focusing on your body, breath, and thoughts is also the concentration for your yoga and meditation practice this week.

As you go through your 40 minute routine each day, bring your focus to the same three things during every part of it.

Body, Breath, and Thoughts ~ Focus and Intention Setting

When you are ready to begin your practice, take two minutes to focus your attention on your body, your breath, and your thoughts - the activity of your mind. You can do this while sitting on the floor or standing, however you feel most comfortable at the time. Please don't worry about being in a lotus position or what you *think* is the proper position for this mindful work. Whatever position is comfortable and allows you to focus inward is perfect.

To begin, take a few moments to notice your body. How do you feel right now in this moment? Sore, tired, invigorated, peaceful?

Now do the same with your breath. What is your breathing like? Notice the gentle pauses between your breaths.

And now your thoughts. Is your mind racing, going over your to do list for the day? Are you revisiting your morning interaction with your husband or kids? Are you worried? Are you content?

You don't have to do anything with what you notice, and remember, this isn't the time to think negatively of yourself. We are simply becoming good at tuning in to where we are in any given moment.

After this, set your intention by asking yourself, "What is it I'm hoping to create in my life by doing this practice today?" Don't rush with your response. Give it a few moments to percolate. Whatever you want to create today doesn't have to be monumental. It's key to start to recognize and acknowledge what you do want to create. That's the first step.

Next, we develop the tools to make that happen. It might seem simple, yet it is very important. It's a way of connecting what we are doing to what we are wanting. And we do this one day at a time.

Notice that the question is about today, not next week or next year. Yes, those bigger and long-term intentions are also important, but for now, let's just look at today. What do you want to create in your life today, and how will this time help you?

MONDAY

Five Minutes

Body, Breath and Thoughts – Focus and Intention Setting upon waking. Focus on the day before you and the intention of your actions.

Thirty Minutes

- Physical activity.

- Take at least five 20-second awareness breaks today.

- Drink 8 glasses of water today.

- Perform one small act today to support your intention of wellness.

- Schedule a treat for yourself later this week.

- Let's do a guided meditation together. Meet me in whatever place and position works best for you.

https://www.youtube.com/watch?v=-LRvhHD82nI&t=7s&ab_channel=CarrieSchell

Today's Thought

Focus on living a quality life.

You are worthy. Treat yourself as though you believe this is true. Commit yourself to living a quality life.

I know that many grey drinkers will read this and think that they do have a quality life. They are accomplished, determined, loved, *happy*. That may be very true. But here's the thing. If there wasn't something: stress, anxiety, depression, insecurity, an inability to unwind, trauma, whatever it may be, then we wouldn't be grey drinking.

Alcohol gives us something. It may help us socialize, relax, make love, chill out, feel good about ourselves, the list goes on. We need to acknowledge that this isn't a healthy way to achieve these things and that we are capable of finding other ways to get there. That is where the true quality of life comes from.

Take advantage of all that is offered to you today. Don't miss a chance to experience beauty in the world and in yourself. Fill yourself with wonder, happiness, and gratitude so you don't have to fill yourself with alcohol.

You deserve a quality life. Treat yourself with kindness and love.

Word for Today: *RELATIONSHIPS*

"Some people come into our lives and leave footprints on our hearts

and we are never ever the same."

~Flavia Weeden

As humans we have a deep need for relationships. As women, we have many types of relationship in our various roles: partner, mother, daughter, sister, friend, colleague.

We all have different kinds of relationships in our lives. Some, we wish we could avoid, while others, it seems, we can never get enough of.

What relationships do you need to nourish in your life? What relationships do you need to set boundaries on? How are your relationships with others going to change over the course of this challenge? What ones will become strengthened and which ones may suffer?

Affirmation

I now enjoy my own company and am becoming an enjoyable companion.

Journaling

Last week you focused on what you were feeding your body and its connection to your drinking. Hopefully you're becoming increasingly aware of how your body is responding to life without alcohol.

This week you will record how your body is responding to the reset. You will record how your body is feeling. Are your cravings lessening at all? How about worrying how this whole challenge is going to play out? How are your heart and mind responding to meditation? Is it challenging, calming, pleasant, troubling? Record it all. Be honest with yourself and express it on the page.

Excerpt

I worry about my mom. I know, I should be focusing on me and not her right now. We are so similar with alcohol. We are both physically active and see that as the permission needed to drink. I think what I find unsettling is how she isn't upfront about it. She actually lies about it. I can honestly say that I am the first to admit that I should cut back or give up drinking for a bit. But she will go through wine and then casually say, "I can't believe how much wine WE went through." And she never goes to bed because she has had too much to drink, but it's always because she's tired. Do you worry about alcohol with someone that age? She is super healthy and yet the whole pattern of it is so troubling.

Exercise

Describe how you've shown up in your different relationships, and what you want to change now.

TUESDAY

Five Minutes

Body, Breath, and Thoughts – Focus and Intention Setting upon waking. Focus on the day before you and the intention of your actions.

Thirty Minutes

- Physical activity.

- Take at least five 20-second awareness breaks today.

- Drink 8 glasses of water today.

- Perform one small act today to support your intention of wellness.

- Schedule a treat for yourself later this week.

- Let's do a guided meditation together. Meet me in whatever place and position works best for you.

https://www.youtube.com/watch?v=S03R-Gxrszg&t=328s&ab_channel=CarrieSchell

Today's Thought

Meditate.

Meditation is foundational to the reset. Maybe you meditate already or maybe this is all new to you. But it is key for nothing else than demonstrating to yourself that you are worthy of these five or ten minutes to heal and honour yourself.

Quiet time is essential to give yourself perspective. Investing in five or ten minutes of silence every day, preferably in the morning before the noise of the day starts, will help ensure your long-term success by keeping you connected to a source of power that lets your weary willpower off the hook.

It will also keep you well grounded, more in charge of your life and more empowered. Mediation, or quiet time, can include prayer, reading spiritual or other uplifting literature, writing in your journal, guided meditations, or simply being in silence. Whatever that looks like for you, allow yourself this gift.

A simple way to begin to meditate on your own is to sit in a comfortable chair, close your eyes, and notice how you are breathing. Pay attention to the air going into your nostrils and going out again. This is simple meditation.

One practice I do is to use a phrase or a few words that I would like to guide my day. It could be something as simple as "happiness" on the inhale and "contentment" on the exhale. When words and thoughts enter your consciousness, simply let them go and resume the focus on your breath.

What you get in return for this simple practice is peace of mind, better health, a more positive attitude, and you'll tap into more love. You also gain a new technique to use, even for a mere two or three minutes, to take time anytime during the day when you need to improve your mood, calm yourself, regroup, and recenter. Some days you will miss your meditation and that's okay. Just try not to miss too many.

This is a gift to yourself. Receive it.

Word for Today: *KINDNESS*

"This is my simple religion. There is no need for temples:

no need for complicated philosophy.

Our own brain, our own heart is our temple; the philosophy is kindness."

~Dalai Lama

True kindness is about being present for others in a positive, nurturing, and loving way without expecting anything in return. Kindness is a type of strength that requires respect for others but also includes emotional affection. Kind people find joy in the act of giving and helping other people, regardless of their degree of relatedness or similarity, and without wanting anything in return.

Affirmation

Kindness is its own reward.

Journaling

How is my body feeling? I can feel my physical body changing already, crazy but true. It feels better, healthier. I love waking up clearheaded, feeling well rested. I have nights when I fall off to sleep easily and others where I lay awake, thinking of a million things and wishing I had a glass of wine to quiet the noise. But I am feeling more confident and good about myself that I am not giving up or giving in. I can do this today. It's just one day. What positive changes are you beginning to notice? Embrace them and honour them by putting them down on paper.

Excerpt

I'm starting to feel good about this not drinking thing. I like the feeling that I am overcoming, that I am growing stronger through this. I do think about how it would be nice to have a drink with dinner, sure, but I also think about how good it felt last night to crawl into bed without having had a drink and keeping true to my intention. I think I can do this.

Exercise

What is the kindest thing someone has done for you?

What is the kindest thing you have ever done for someone else?

WEDNESDAY

Five Minutes

Body, Breath, and Thoughts – Focus and Intention Setting upon waking. Focus on the day before you and the intention of your actions.

Thirty Minutes

- Physical activity.

- Take at least five 20-second awareness breaks today.

- Drink 8 glasses of water today.

- Perform one small act today to support your intention of wellness.

- Schedule a treat for yourself later this week.

- Let's do a guided meditation together. Meet me in whatever place and position works best for you.

https://www.youtube.com/watch?v=OTzP3a_50T4&t=10s&ab_channel=CarrieSchell

Today's Thought

Include an awareness of Spirit.

If you feel that you need to make a change with your drinking, please open your mind to the possibility that an awareness of Spirit may have been something previously missing or neglected in your life. For many, connecting with a higher power is key in letting go of alcohol in their lives.

I believe it is essential to realize that there is more to you than your accomplishments, wealth, beauty, or number of likes on Instagram. There is light within you, our higher, deeper, or true self that is this spiritual part of you, your essence.

When we give ourselves permission to allow awareness in and accept that there is great beauty and love within us, we are more likely to nurture and support ourselves. When you own this, you're more likely to live a healthy life because you value yourself more fully and you'll have something more than your human willpower to depend on.

How does that happen? When you begin to acknowledge your higher self, your self-worth develops and intuitively guides you toward healthier, more supportive practices. You begin to care. And now, for the first time in a long time, that person you are caring about is you.

Going deeper and having a spiritual component is absolutely necessary if you believe you've done all you can to get a grip on your grey drinking and it keeps getting harder, and not easier, over time. If you can't do this yourself, give yourself a break and turn it over to something that can, whatever Higher Power that is for you.

Including a spiritual component is simply knowing when you're up against something that is too much for you and your best intentions to handle on your own. It's realizing when you need to depend on something that is beyond our physical self, whether you think of that as God, nature, or a power that, although beyond your human ego, resides in yourself.

Word for Today: *GRIEF*

"Substance abuse treatment is a fertile field for dealing with the grief process. Patients and their families present for treatment grieving the loss of the mood-altering substance, the loss of vitality, the loss of a family, the loss of employment, the loss of youth, the loss of self-respect, and for many, the loss of spirituality. But few are aware of this. Like most, they don't associate substance abuse treatment with any form of grief."

~Kenneth A. Lucas, *A Buddhist Approach to Addiction, Grief, and Psychotherapy*

Think of it this way: our substance was our best "frenemy." It was always there for us - whatever the mood, whatever the situation, we could always rely on our substance to be there, going through life with us. In some fucked-up way, we depended on our substance rather than depending on others, or ourselves, to get us through life. But where did it really leave us in the end?

It's normal to fear what life will be like without it. How could you not have fear? For so long this "thing" has been your steadfast companion, your partner in crime. Your alcohol has become part of you to define you. Take away the alcohol, what does that leave? It can be really hard to even remember what you were truly like before all of this started.

Be kind to yourself. You are not failing because you worry how you will stop drinking. It is normal to worry and to be afraid. Actually, this is a necessary stage of the journey. Just trust and know you will develop new patterns, new strategies, new coping skills, and real relationships that support and nurture you, rather than deplete your mind, body, and spirit.

Affirmation

I now choose the simple pleasures of everyday living.

Journaling

My grey drinking crept up on me over the years. It was so sneaky that I didn't even realize it at first.

The crazy thing is that in my "professional" life, I was the Director of Health and Wellness at a residential addiction centre and I was good at it, really good. I helped many people navigate through their life of addiction and alcoholism. And yet privately, I would go home and unwind from an incredibly trying day, yet rewarding day at the centre, with a glass or two of wine. I could hear a little voice telling me how crazy that was, helping people stop drinking by day and yet using alcohol to unwind at night.

Excerpt

It is so helpful to just think about. I know, I know, I've heard it, I've actually said it to clients before…but thinking about today and understanding and appreciating that I have enough grace, strength, and resolve for today is a gift. I can make it through today, and tomorrow's today. I can. I have been. It is getting easier. I am feeling lighter. It's becoming less of a burden.

Exercise

Write to your drinking with all your feelings and memories. Tell your drinking everything, both good and bad. Allow yourself to experience all of the emotions this brings up for you. This is a powerful process.

THURSDAY

Five Minutes

Body, Breath, and Thoughts – Focus and Intention Setting upon waking. Focus on the day before you and the intention of your actions.

Thirty Minutes

- Physical activity.

- Take at least five 20-second awareness breaks today.

- Drink 8 glasses of water today.

- Perform one small act today to support your intention of wellness.

- Schedule a treat for yourself later this week.

- Let's do a guided meditation together. Meet me in whatever place and position works best for you.

https://www.youtube.com/watch?v=deH14yUg5Q4&ab_channel=CarrieSchell

Today's Thought

Stay centered in today.

This whole notion of being centered in today is super important to your success. Our overall goal is to not be a grey drinker, right? But we need to take baby steps.

Our grey drinking didn't happen overnight. It took its gentle, clever time to wield its way into our lives and establish itself as a key player. And so, it is going to take time to remove its importance to us.

This is where the staying centered comes in. Today we are not going to drink. We are only going to think about today. We are not going to worry about what we will do at the wedding that's coming up next month. We won't worry about what it looks like to hang out with friends we used to have drinks with. We are going to focus on today. We are granted strength for one day and today, so today you've got it covered. Real change occurs with time. Small changes will add up. It's those small changes that will create a significant change in your life.

Stay centered in today. You can do it.

Staying centered in the now keeps you focused on what you are doing. When you stay focused, you fully experience the day, its events, its sensations, and the growth you're experiencing. Life will become richer and more gratifying. You will worry less because worry is about the future. When the future becomes the present, it won't be nearly as frightening.

An added incentive for staying in today is that this is where everything is happening: life, pleasure and your successes. Today is life. Today is your moment.

Word for Today: *MEDITATION*

"We now realize that it (meditation) activates the prefrontal cortex – the seat of higher thinking, and stimulates the release of neurotransmitters, including dopamine, serotonin, oxytocin, and brain opiates. Each of these naturally occurring brain chemicals has been linked to different aspects of happiness. Dopamine is an antidepressant, serotonin is associated with increased self-esteem, oxytocin is now believed to be the pleasant hormone, and opiates are the body's painkillers. No single drug can simultaneously choreograph the coordinated release of all of these chemicals."

~Deepak Chopra, *The Ultimate Happiness Prescription*

In today's world, how do we create a healthy balance between material success and externals with internal joy and peace? It's tough. All of our messaging is geared towards what we have, how we look, and how many "likes" we get.

How do we navigate our inner turmoil and challenges when everyone else appears to have it so together with perfect smiles and perfect pictures? Where do we get to be vulnerable and honest and let go of the facades? How can we possibly have a perfect marriage, perfect kids, perfect job, and perfect body? I don't think it is possible.

But one thing I do know is that meditation and yoga can help. They won't change your circumstances, but they will change you how view your circumstances. They act as a rudder, helping to navigate rough waters and find internal peace and calm.

Affirmation

I find peace within.

Journaling

What do you do if your partner is a grey drinker also? How is that going to impact your success with the reset? Are they willing to do the reset? Do they acknowledge that they are a grey drinker? Have they expressed they'd like to stop drinking? How has alcohol impacted your relationship? How is not drinking alcohol going to impact your relationship?

Excerpt

My husband thinks I don't know, but I do. I know the things he does, how could I possibly not? That's the crazy part. He actually thinks I don't clue into what he's doing. Buying a litre bottle of wine so that he can drink more than one bottle in an evening but it doesn't seem like it because there is still quite a bit left. Having a margarita and switching to wine because that makes it look like he isn't drinking as many drinks. Asking me out to lunch to have a drink or two during the day. I know all the tricks. I call him on them. He's not ready to let the drinking go. But he's getting there.

Exercise

Choose to dedicate ten minutes every morning and every night to breathing deeply and calmly while repeating the affirmation, "I find peace within." Take time to reflect and capture in your journal how you feel, mind, body and spirit afterwards.

FRIDAY

Five Minutes

Body, Breath, and Thoughts – Focus and Intention Setting upon waking. Focus on the day before you and the intention of your actions.

Thirty Minutes

- Physical activity.

- Take at least five 20-second awareness breaks today.

- Drink 8 glasses of water today.

- Perform one small act today to support your intention of wellness.

- Schedule a treat for yourself later this week.

- Let's do a guided meditation together. Meet me in whatever place and position works best for you.

https://www.youtube.com/watch?v=FpLp7waxoNU&ab_channel=CarrieSchell

Today's Thought

You are always more than enough.

Remember, perfection does not exist in this world and sometimes you will struggle. This program does not prevent life from happening. You will continue to live, laugh, and even hurt. This is part of the process.

Set reasonable parameters for yourself. Go into this day with the honest intention of contentment, moving forward, and not dwelling on past wrongs. You are always more than enough.

Word for Today: *RECOVERY*

"I believe that if we are truly to recover from the disease of addiction, we must grow emotionally. True recovery is the product of humility that emerges from living and practicing a conscious and spiritual life. In order to attain humility, we must be honest with ourselves. This necessarily includes looking at the stupid things we do, today, in recovery. I use the term stupid to indicate the things we do that are self-destructive and not in our best interest."

~Allen Berger, *12 Stupid Things That Mess Up Recovery*

Recovery is the first step of the rest of our lives. We have the ultimate freedom of choice, and it is important to begin with this understanding. We are not victims, regardless of how powerless we felt in the depths of our grey drinking. You have now reclaimed your life. Honour your power to make this choice permanent. Recovery is always your choice.

Affirmation

I choose recovery.

Journaling

Wondering and worrying how letting go of drinking will impact your friendships is valid. Not all of your friends are going to be supportive or even like the fact that you aren't drinking. Some will playfully pour you a drink and tell you that you don't need to worry, you're not an alcoholic.

No, you're not an alcoholic but that doesn't mean that your drinking hasn't wandered into grey territories. I have friends that I love dearly, but realize that when we get together, we *always* drink. Always. We don't go on hikes or walks. I don't do anything physically active with them. Our socializing is always centered on drinking.

I don't know how stopping drinking is going to impact our friendship. I pray there is something deeper there than alcohol. And yet, maybe, just maybe, my stopping drinking will give them the courage and support they need to change their drinking behaviours. But honestly, I can't even dwell on that. I need to nurture me right now. Put the oxygen mask on yourself before helping others.

Excerpt

I was alone this evening and bought a bag of chips to snack on. I don't know why because I'm trying not to eat junk right now and cleanse my body. But seeing as I'm not drinking and I wanted a little treat, I bought the stupid chips. I ate the whole bag. It wasn't a big bag, but still. I hate not feeling in control. I felt gross and sick. Good lesson. I think I want something, but really, I don't.

Exercise

Remind yourself of all the good reasons you have chosen to be present in your life.

SATURDAY

Five Minutes

Body, Breath, and Thoughts – Focus and Intention Setting upon waking. Focus on the day before you and the intention of your actions.

Thirty Minutes

- Physical activity.

- Take at least five 20-second awareness breaks today.

- Drink 8 glasses of water today.

- Perform one small act today to support your intention of wellness.

- Schedule a treat for yourself later this week.

- Let's do a guided meditation together. Meet me in whatever place and position works best for you.

https://www.youtube.com/watch?v=-HhSnob0DUw&ab_channel=CarrieSchell

Today's Thought

Give your senses something to do.

Our senses help keep us alive and help us appreciate that we are in the here and now. We need to nurture our senses by taking the time to appreciate the beauty and richness all around us, in its many forms.

Take a few moments to feel blessed when taking in a beautiful sunset, or the sound of laughter, or the loving hug of a friend.

Eyes like seeing beauty, colour, and the joys of life. Ears like hearing lovely music, lyrical words, and the voices of people who care for them. Skin and nerve endings and the muscles underneath long for touch and stimulation. The olfactory nerves that detect smells also carry us back to some of the best moments of our lives.

When living under the haze of alcohol, our senses become dulled, not fully alive. Things don't taste the same. Music is not the same. Even movies and television become background noise.

As the days progress, take time to reawaken your senses. Look at the colours that surround you. Enjoy the smells coming from the kitchen where your meals are cooking. Allow your muscles to come alive during yoga. Sink into the sounds of your early morning body, breath, and thoughts.

Indulge in all of your senses.

Word for Today: *SELF-ESTEEM*

"True self-esteem is not the same thing as improving your self-image. Self-image results from what other people think of you. The true self lies beyond images. It can be found at a level of existence that is independent of the good and bad opinions of others. It is fearless. It has infinite worth. When you shift your identity from your self-image to your true self, you will find happiness that no one can take away from you."

~Deepak Chopra, *The Ultimate Happiness Prescription*

Self-esteem is earned through our thoughts, words, and deeds. It's not easy to learn to value our true self based on who we are, rather than what we have or do. The enduring qualities and virtues of a life well lived are created by our own doing.

If you were blessed with good parents that helped create within you a healthy sense of self-worth, that's wonderful. But it's only as adults that we can decide if we like the person looking back in the mirror. The truth will always come back from a deep place within: the inner self that cannot lie no matter how hard our ego tries to practice self-deception.

Affirmation

I will strive to be honorable in my thoughts, words, and deeds.

Journaling

Have you ever gone on a diet and once you start all you can think about is food? Seriously. Am I the only one who, when that Monday rolls around, am famished and craving food to eat that I haven't eaten in weeks or months.

Our mind is a powerful thing. We may have all the desires, intentions, and heaps of willpower, but man, once you give up drinking, it can be an all-consuming thought – especially when we are doing a 30-day reset that asks us to think about drinking each and every day.

But here's the thing. There must be a part of you, at some point during this journey, that is feeling pretty friggin' good about sticking with the challenge this far. When you start longing for a margarita on the rocks with a salted rim, allow yourself the gift of remembering how good those moments felt. Remember why you began the reset. Remember how good you know you are going to feel when you stop wondering if you drink too much and if it is normal to drink this much. It will be freeing, liberating. Each day thus far has given you that gift. Lean into it and accept it in its entirety.

Excerpt

Lovemaking is better when no one has had a drink. Way better. It is so much more intentional, focused. It feels better and everything is heightened. Beyond the physical, the intimacy is far greater.

This is a good thing. Remember this.

Exercise

Imagine what you will feel when you feel good about yourself. How will your life be different?

SUNDAY

If you have already completed the previous six days this week, then this day is a free day to spend an hour doing something that you really love to do.

This is your second weekend that you are on the reset, and it is most likely pretty tough.

Have you passed on going out for dinner or brunch today to avoid refusing that glass of bubbly or having to explain that you're doing this reset? If you have, it's okay. You are doing what you need to do to take care of you in this early stage of the journey.

You may find that your friends and family are super supportive. You may even want to ask some of them if they want to join you on the challenge. Getting support from others is important. This is a very courageous thing that you're doing, seriously. How many people do you know who may be grey drinkers are taking those first steps to make change and empower themselves? So proud of you.

If you've missed a day, why don't you honour yourself and hunker down and do it. You are so worth it. Enjoy a guided meditation.

Here's the link for the Sunday meditation: https://www.youtube.com/watch?v=AGXHWm7rVoQ&ab_channel=CarrieSchell

Please accept this gift I am offering you.

Week 3

The theme for this week is acceptance. Last week we practiced becoming more aware. Now it's time to learn how to accept whatever awareness comes to us.

Practicing acceptance does not mean that you are surrendering to the status quo and are not going to change anything. It simply means you are accepting what is, opening your heart and mind to change.

The steps of becoming aware and then learning to accept what we have discovered about ourselves are often not part of life's process. These steps take both time and self-inquiry. It's easier to skip these steps and rush towards the first possible solution that appears.

Or maybe we don't even slow down enough to develop awareness. We just keep going, full speed ahead, hoping for change but never doing the work to make change happen. I'm asking you to avoid the need to find a solution immediately. Stop rushing and trust in the Universe, God, your higher power, whatever you are rooted in. Have acceptance in whatever you discover about yourself on this journey.

What if I Can't Accept?

You may have already asked that question. If you haven't, I can assure you that if you follow the guidance on practicing acceptance this week, there will be times when doubts arise.

You will probably come across a particular awareness that you don't feel you can accept or even just let be. What do you do with that?

Well, the answer is simple, kind of. Just notice yourself not being able to accept. That is part of your reality, part of your awareness of self, and like everything else, it can be accepted also.

Your program this week is similar to what you did last week with a few minor variations to fit the theme of acceptance.

Noticing and Accepting ~ Focus and Intention Setting

This week, as you begin your daily practice, take a few minutes to focus on acceptance. Do this by first focusing on your body. Notice and accept it just the way it is.

Do the same with your breath and whatever else you are noticing about yourself as you begin your practice.

Also, take a moment to bring to your awareness what it is you want to create in your life. Spend this time today to set your intention.

Meditation

Use our meditation this week to practice acceptance. Accept any thought you notice. Accept any drifting into your past or future.

A little trick you can use to help with practicing acceptance as you meditate is to notice and then simply say to yourself, "And it is so." Exhale as you do.

Journaling

This week, make the focus of your journal writing your awareness of yourself around the theme of acceptance.

What can you accept about yourself? What is difficult to accept? What guidance did you receive about this and how might it apply to your life?

Record anything else of importance that you notice either during your practice or in the rest of your day.

At this point in our journey, you will probably notice behaviours in yourself and others that you were oblivious to before. This can bring up many things, both positive and negative.

Right now, be aware of what you are experiencing but don't try to find solutions. Take a "Huh, I never noticed that before," attitude.

It is very challenging, but being able to develop this practice will benefit you tremendously in the upcoming days and weeks.

Awareness Breaks

During the day this week and in subsequent weeks, take some 20-second awareness breaks. *An awareness break is simply stopping what you are doing or thinking or saying and being still for 20 seconds.*

Use those 20 seconds to notice what is happening to you and around you. One thing I absolutely love to do, especially if I am on a hike or out somewhere being active, is to simply stop, close my eyes, and stand still for 20 seconds. It is incredible how an awareness of peace and calm is experienced. Try it. You don't have to be hiking. Do it at your desk at work or standing in the kitchen, or on the subway. It's a very cool practice.

MONDAY

Two Minutes

Notice and Accepting ~ Focus and Intention Setting

Five Minutes

- Take at least five 20-second awareness breaks today.

- Practice accepting all that you notice.

- Perform one small act to support your intention.

- Schedule a treat for your body later this week.

Thirty Minutes

- Physical activity and enjoy a guided meditation.

- Drink 8 glasses of water today

- Let's do a guided meditation together. Meet me in whatever place and position works best for you.

https://www.youtube.com/watch?v=-LRvhHD82nI&t=7s&ab_channel=CarrieSchell

Today's Thought

Deal with your stress.

This is your opportunity to learn new methods for dealing with life's stressors.

There are tons of ways to reduce stress and we'll explore ways to do that together – and find what works best for you.

Learning yoga and meditation, getting regular exercise, seeing a therapist, or looking more closely at what spirituality has to offer, are all great stress reduction techniques.

The journaling you're doing also helps with this. If you have a person you trust, that makes you feel safe, try talking about your problems and decisions with them. But be sure it is someone who will listen more than talk.

There are other techniques that can be readily used. The easiest and most available is breathing. We've already explored breathing in the previous weeks, but it is such a simple, effective tool, that I wanted to go over it again.

Slow, deep breathing ~ in through your nose, out through your mouth ~ can calm you down when you are anxious or angry.

A hot bath will work.

Self-massage ~ kneading the kinks out of your shoulders, neck, and hands can help reduce tension.

A change of scene ~ go outside if you're inside, lie down if you're up, take a walk if you are vegging on the couch.

Begin to recognize which situations cause stress in your life and can be triggers to relapse. Recognizing these situations goes a long way in both preventing and managing your life and having more control and ownership.

Alcohol is what you used to use to get you through, or avoid, experiencing stress. Now you've got to figure out how to get through the tough times without something that may have *served* you for a long time. You need to replace it with other tools.

I'm not going to sugarcoat it for you. This is incredibly challenging. But, if you are willing to try to begin to deal with stress in healthy ways, you will eventually live a life fuller and happier than what you're experiencing now. You'll live a happier life rooted in wellness.

Word for Today: *SELF-DISCOVERY*

"When you take the first step towards self-development,
many doors of friendship and happiness will be opened for you."

~Unknown

Many addictions are caused by the fear of one's own inner self. We don't want to deal with painful or uncomfortable emotions, so we try to suppress, ignore, drown, or change the way we feel through substances. We now know that doesn't work.

Self-discovery means turning our attention inward and exploring who you are. This is no small feat because it's uncharted territory with no map to guide us.

So what exactly does self-discovery mean? Self-discovery means paying attention and discovering who you are. Self-discovery means that we are responsible for being aware of our needs and how to nurture our true self.

Affirmation

I am now willing to embark on the voyage of self-discovery.

Journaling

This week, make the focus of your journal writing your awareness of yourself around the theme of acceptance.

Record anything else of importance that you notice either during your practice or in the rest of your day.

Excerpt

I think I was able to connect and relate to people at the addiction centre and truly help them in their recovery because I had addicts and alcoholics that I loved in my life. I knew them. I understood them.

I also had the understanding and awareness of what it was like to be the child of that person, or the wife, or the sister. I got it. I got what made them tick and yet, that wasn't me. That wasn't my truth. I never lied or misled clients into believing that I was in recovery. But in a weird way, I was on that journey with them. It wasn't until I heard the expression "grey drinking" that it clicked. I knew right then and there that is what I was. There was no questioning. There was no need to Google and do research. That was it. I finally had a label, a name for my alcohol consumption – grey drinking.

Exercise

Talk about yourself.

What's your favorite music? What food do you love? How about hobbies or sports? What makes you really happy? What pisses you off?

Start simple. Write down what you do know about yourself. What's your favorite music? What food do you love? How about hobbies or sports? What makes you really happy? What annoys the hell out of you?

TUESDAY

Two Minutes

Notice and Accepting ~ Focus and Intention Setting

Five Minutes

- Take at least five 20-second awareness breaks today.

- Practice accepting all that you notice.

- Perform one small act to support your intention.

Thirty Minutes

- Physical activity.

- Drink 8 glasses of water today.

- Let's do a guided meditation together. Proud of you.

https://www.youtube.com/watch?v=S03R-Gxrszg&t=328s&ab_channel=CarrieSchell

Today's Thought

Be kind to yourself on difficult days.

Everyone has to deal with bad days. It's not magic – you get through them by going through them.

The challenge for someone struggling with not drinking is how to get through bad days without giving into the temptation to drink. To do this, you first have to resign yourself to the fact that difficult days are normal and happen to everyone, even to people who seem to have a perfect life.

The next step is to remind yourself, as often as necessary, that in almost every case, shitty times are temporary. It's completely normal when you're at this point to see every difficulty as permanent. Don't worry. You're not alone in feeling this way.

To keep from drinking, it is important that you recognize the difference between a bad day and a futile life. Once you realize you are having a bad day or two, you can take a moment and give yourself a break, cut yourself some slack, and treat yourself to an act of kindness. ***This is when you need to learn to be gentle with yourself and practice this gentleness when it means the most.***

It is also important to acknowledge that we may have more than one bad day. During stretches that seem really rough, you have to intentionally put something bright into each day, even if you think it would feel better to be miserable.

This is easier said than done, I know. But I promise that if you make the effort to support yourself with kindness, it will be returned to you tenfold.

Spiritual readings are likely to speak to you more clearly now than at any other time. You'll even find new insights in readings familiar to you. If you feel you are in real trouble, you need to seek someone out: a counselor, a spiritual leader, whoever, and acknowledge your struggles without losing sight of all that is full of hope and goodness.

Word for Today: *FREEDOM*

"Freedom is nothing else but a chance to be better."

~Albert Camus

"No man is free who in not a master of himself."

~Epicteus

Liberty, autonomy, lack of restrictions, self-determination, independence, choice, and free-will are some of the synonyms for this wondrous state of being. You are now well into your own freedom from the chains of alcohol that were controlling your life.

History shows how fiercely we fight to be free – countless brave people have sacrificed their lives in the name of freedom. Are you willing to sacrifice your freedom anymore?

Affirmation

I have the courage to fight for my freedom from addiction to drinking.

Journaling

This week, make the focus of your journal writing your awareness of yourself around the theme of acceptance.

"What can I accept about myself? What is difficult to accept? What guidance did I receive about this and how might it apply to my life?"

Record anything else of importance that you notice either during your practice or in the rest of your day.

Excerpt

See, this is how your mind starts messing with you. If I could cut back, if I could have a healthy relationship with alcohol, why wouldn't I have that already? Why wouldn't I just cut back? Why would I miss it when I don't have wine at night?

Because I can't. I have no idea if that will ever change. I don't know if grey drinkers are able to ever just have a glass of wine. This is a whole new area and there isn't much out there on this.

But right now, I know that I cannot drink. There is no cutting back for me. I have to just not drink. That's it. And I have to be okay with that.

Exercise

"The basic test of freedom is perhaps less in what we are free to do

than in what we are not free to do."

~Eric Hoffler

Describe how it's beginning to feel as you become free of your need to drink. Describe the battles it took to make this decision.

WEDNESDAY

Two Minutes

Notice and Accepting ~ Focus and Intention Setting

Five Minutes

- Take at least five 20-second awareness breaks today.

- Practice accepting all that you notice.

- Perform one small act to support your intention.

- Schedule a treat for your body later this week.

Thirty Minutes

- Physical activity.

- Drink 8 glasses of water today.

- Let's do a guided meditation together. Proud of you.

https://www.youtube.com/watch?v=OTzP3a_50T4&t=10s&ab_channel=CarrieSchell

Today's Thought

Develop an attitude of gratitude.

Have an attitude of gratitude. Without an attitude of gratitude, renewable every day, you leave yourself open to negativity and that is often the first step to uncorking that bottle. Acknowledging your blessings with gratitude is key to preventing drinking.

A helpful exercise is to write ten things you're grateful for every day in your journal. If you get discouraged, frustrated, or overwhelmed during the day, write ten more. Big things, little things, it doesn't matter. They can even be the same ten things every day.

Once you acknowledge and write your ten gratitudes, your day looks different. Your life feels better. Your world seems more accommodating.

On tough mornings, the ones when getting out of bed seems like a bad idea, you may want to make your list mentally before your feet touch the floor. It can get your priorities in order almost instantly.

When gratitude moves in, happiness usually comes along. If you start every day by making a gratitude list, whether on paper or in your mind and heart, you are consciously aware that you are living a life worthy of gratitude and life becomes that much sweeter.

You are then able to acknowledge the good things that happen to you during your day. Things you may have overlooked before now become blessings. You'll notice beauty you may have overlooked before. Eventually you will find it hard to keep your list to ten.

Word for Today: *FOCUS*

How often has someone said to you, "Would you please just focus?" How do we train ourselves to remain focused on one subject at a time?

The answer is simple. It is known as mindfulness.

Pay attention to the present moment, be mindful of everything around you, and most importantly, stop time traveling in your mind. The majority of people are living in the past, thinking about the future, scattered everywhere in their mind except in the only place that truly exists – this present moment. Focus helps you constantly correct your course. Staying in the present moment and taking good care of what is before you are refreshing.

Your brain is just like a muscle. You are able to exercise being in the moment with practice and mindfulness. Start by becoming aware of when you are thinking of things from the past or things yet to come. Next, notice how often you are doing this. Slowly start to acknowledge those thoughts and bring your mind back to the present, to today.

Affirmation

I am mindful. I am focused.

Journaling

This week, make the focus of your journal writing your awareness of yourself around the theme of acceptance.

"What can I accept about myself? What is difficult to accept? What guidance did I receive about this and how might it apply to my life?"

Record anything else of importance that you notice either during your practice or in the rest of your day.

Excerpt

I am starting to lose weight. I am starting to feel lighter. My cheekbones are taking on shape, definition. I am losing the bloating in my belly. My ass hasn't gotten any smaller, this isn't a miracle worker, but I am feeling better. I like how I am feeling. I am encouraged by how I am feeling. Something positive is coming from this and that is sooo good. And that is enough to be thankful for and to motivate me for tomorrow. I am changing and for the better.

Exercise

An excellent tool in retraining your mind is memorizing something simple. It allows you to concentrate and focus your attention on the present.

Try to memorize the saying below. Go on, give it a shot.

"We are what we think.
All that we are arises with our thoughts.
With our thoughts, we make our world."
~Buddha

Try to write about how easy or difficult it was to memorize this passage. How hard is it for you to let go of the past and stop turning your thoughts to the future? How could being present in today benefit you?

THURSDAY

Two Minutes

Notice and Accepting ~ Focus and Intention Setting

Five Minutes

- Take at least five 20-second awareness breaks today.

- Practice accepting all that you notice.

- Perform one small act to support your intention.

- Schedule a treat for your body later this week.

Thirty Minutes

- Physical activity.

- Drink 8 glasses of water today.

- Let's do a guided meditation together. Proud of you.

https://www.youtube.com/watch?v=deH14yUg5Q4&ab_channel=CarrieSchell

Today's Thought

Just keep moving forward.

Changing from the inside means making changes in both how you live and think. This is why I encourage you to explore the many varied and rich aspects of your being.

How you see yourself, how you relate to the world around you, and how much help you are willing to accept from whatever higher power is part of your sense of things, are all key to this self-exploration. You will realize you are more than the person you were when your drinking became unhealthy and you began to take on more negative thoughts and behaviors.

Even when everything is coming together, I still want you to keep your focus on today, taking small steps forward. Do whatever you need to do to keep from drinking. Do not think in terms of tomorrow or forever. Today is enough.

Use techniques you are learning. Be fearless in your desire to succeed by reaching out to those who will help you. You can expect to get what you need, including the transformation to make the most of your life.

Perfection does not exist in this world, and sometimes you will be tempted to drink. Of course, you will. You will remember drinking almost romantically. This is part of the process. It's how you learn that life without alcohol is enough. Your life without alcohol has value and meaning.

Go into this day with the honest intention of staying committed to the journey you're on. Keep moving forward today and leave the past behind.

Word for the Day: PATIENCE

"One moment of patience may ward off great disaster.

One moment of impatience may ruin a whole life."

~Chinese proverb

"Patience is also a form of action."

~August Robin

"Adopt the pace of nature: her secret is patience."

~Ralph Waldo Emerson

I felt that this was the perfect place for this word, patience. Nearing the end of week three, you've been working the program, being mindful, and cultivating new awarenesses.

Unlike other "programs," developing a healthy relationship with alcohol doesn't have a clear finish line. The further along we progress, (and yes, we are progressing), the harder it can be.

We are becoming clearer that alcohol isn't serving a purpose, but we're also becoming clearer on why we have leaned on alcohol, why we needed this source of apparent strength outside of ourselves.

And so, patience. Be patient with yourself. Know that because you are still experiencing challenging moments, thoughts and relationships, doesn't mean it isn't worth the journey. You are perfectly imperfect and that is always more than enough.

Affirmation

Patience is waiting.

Patience is not passively waiting. That is laziness. But to keep going when the going is hard and slow – this is patience.

Journaling

This week, make the focus of your journal writing your awareness of yourself around the theme of acceptance.

"What can I accept about myself? What is difficult to accept? What guidance did I receive about this and how might it apply to my life?"

Record anything else of importance that you notice either during your practice or in the rest of your day.

Excerpt

It is so fucking annoying that I can be so disciplined and organized and keep it all really together, juggling so much, and I let this one thing get to this point? Why can't I just be normal and not want enjoy wine so much? How is it that I have friends who eat like crap, never exercise, but couldn't care less if they ever have a drink? How does that work? How is it that me, who puts effort into being fit and healthy, also likes to have a couple of glasses of wine at night? Why do I find it so hard to let it go? It just doesn't make sense to my rational self. Ugh. I am so annoying.

Exercise

Explore how patience is essential in recovery. How has not having patience derailed you in the past?

FRIDAY

Two Minutes

Notice and Accepting ~ Focus and Intention Setting

Five Minutes

- Take at least five 20-second awareness breaks today.

- Practice accepting all that you notice.

- Perform one small act to support your intention.

- Schedule a treat for your body later this week.

Thirty Minutes

- Physical activity.

- Drink 8 glasses of water today.

- Let's do a guided meditation together. Proud of you.

https://www.youtube.com/watch?v=FpLp7waxoNU&ab_channel=CarrieSchell

Today's Thought

Make peace with your past and other people.

The past is over, but it is not necessarily done with. Until it is, it can lead to a return to drinking. Wading in old hurts and disappointments is never easy, but without being willing to face the deep-seated issues that may be responsible or contributing to your drinking, you may be keeping yourself in a vulnerable place, and risking your life without alcohol.

An effective way to make peace is to forgive the people who harmed you and forgive yourself for your own mistakes. Deal with the instances in which you feel you were at fault by showing up and setting things right to the degree that you can. Then, you have to let it go. If letting go is hard for you, keep at it. It's hard for everybody, but it is essential to your well-being.

When someone has hurt you, forgiveness can be challenging. To be perfectly clear, forgiveness is not saying, "It's okay that you were terrible to me. You can do it again."

Rather, it's realizing that hurt comes from hurt. Forgiveness releases the person to their own fate, and frees you from the old hurts. This is equally important if you're in need of forgiving yourself from the harm you have caused yourself, and others.

Don't kid yourself, your act of forgiveness is as much for you as for the other person. You need the weight of what happened lifted from your heart and mind. What you have done does not define who you are. At your core, you are truly a source of light and love.

Do the work that needs to be done. Seek out the help and guidance you need from a friend, family member, professional, or spiritual mentor. The guidance of someone else may enable you to experience a series of *aha* moments so things that never made sense before can start becoming clear.

Value yourself and this process enough to make peace with yourself and others.

Word for Today: *INNER WISDOM*

Where does wisdom come from?

Wisdom speaks from all corners of our world, and age is not always a factor. Wisdom comes from a calm knowingness, life experience, a clear and sober mind, and an ability to see the bigger picture.

Understanding, knowledge, insight, perception, astuteness, intelligence, acumen, and good judgement are all synonyms for wisdom. Your decision to begin this wellness journey is a wise decision. You have wisdom within you. Do not lose sight of this and listen to your inner voice, your inner truth. Begin to trust this inner voice, your inner wisdom. It is your guide.

Affirmation

I now choose to cultivate wisdom in all life choices.

Journaling

This week, make the focus of your journal writing your awareness of yourself around the theme of acceptance.

"What can I accept about myself? What is difficult to accept? What guidance did I receive about this and how might it apply to my life?"

Record anything else of importance that you notice either during your practice or in the rest of your day.

Excerpt

I have tried many times to take a break from drinking. I have set deadlines, had countdowns, and yet it never sticks.

I have thought that if only I try harder, get more determined, dig down deep and get some will power, I will be able to do it.

And so I am handing it all over. I am laying it down and just asking God to help me on this one. I don't want to be the kind of person that relies on alcohol. I want to be the person that realized she depended on alcohol and gave it up and became a better woman for it.

I want to inspire my kids. I want them to see I can do it. I want to see I can do it. I want to help other women do it also. I can't be the only one out there struggling with this.

I want to help others…

Exercise

Think carefully of all the times you have made a wise decision. List the benefits you enjoyed from this.

SATURDAY

Two Minutes

Notice and Accepting ~ Focus and Intention Setting

Five Minutes

- Take at least five 20-second awareness breaks today.

- Practice accepting all that you notice.

- Perform one small act to support your intention.

- Schedule a treat for your body later this week.

Thirty Minutes

- Physical activity.

- Drink 8 glasses of water today.

- Let's do a guided meditation together. The light in me honours the light in you.

https://www.youtube.com/watch?v=-HhSnob0DUw&ab_channel=CarrieSchell

Today's Thought

It's all going to be okay. Our challenging times are preparing us for the next great thing.

One thing I have come to truly believe is that, when we are going through truly shitty times, the universe is readying us for the next phase we are about to enter. Having that knowing is both a comfort and strength. I still have times in my life when I disappoint myself tremendously or relationships are experiencing true hardships. But now, I am able to actually step back and know the hardships will pass.

You don't have to appear as though you have it all under control every minute of the day. It is essential to refuse to worry about what you cannot do anything about. Do your best to be less distraught when things don't work out the way you hoped they would. More often than not, this means that life has something better in store for you anyhow.

Sometimes we just need to trust that our challenging periods happen to prepare and strengthen us for the good that is in store for us. When you begin to place your trust and hope in God and the universe and when you begin to believe it will all work out even though you cannot see a possible way, know that you carry a light within you.

It is the light of hope, goodness, and love, and it radiates outward. Your light instills hope in others, and encourages them on their journey, through their struggles.

Word for Today: *COMPASSION*

Most people think of compassion as an admirable character trait like honesty, loyalty, or spontaneity. If you have compassion, you show it by being kind, sympathetic and helpful to others. This is definitely true.

But here's the thing. Compassion, like self esteem, is not an unchanging character trait. Compassion is actually a skill; a skill that you can increase if you lack it or improve it if you already have it. And compassion is not something you feel only for others. It should also inspire you to be kind, sympathetic and helpful to yourself. There are three basic attributes that make up compassion: understanding, acceptance, and forgiveness.

Affirmation

As a compassionate person, I am now kind,
sympathetic, and helpful to myself and others.

Journaling

This week, make the focus of your journal writing your awareness of yourself around the theme of acceptance.

"What can I accept about myself? What is difficult to accept? What guidance did I receive about this and how might it apply to my life?"

Record anything else of importance that you notice either during your practice or in the rest of your day.

Excerpt

I feel like I am the foundation of our family. That sounds boastful, but in a way, I do. I feel like the glue that keeps the parts together and connected.

I created and keep all of the family traditions for holidays, birthdays, everything. I love doing it. The happiest times of my life are when we are all together, but sometimes, just sometimes, I want to be the one who gets taken care of.

I don't want to spend hours and days cooking and cleaning for a holiday only to miss a lot of it making sure everyone has what they need and treating them to a special time. I'm not complaining, and I wouldn't change it for anything, but sometimes...

Maybe that is how I relax through those holidays and times we're together. I know it's definitely the way I was brought up to host those times. Lots of food, drinks, desserts, music, dancing, laughter.

Offering a drink when someone arrives is second nature. I can't imagine not doing that because I am not drinking. But how do I make it not weird and uncomfortable for everyone else?

Exercise

Write how learning the skill of compassion could change the way you treat yourself and others. Choose a positive memory when someone treated you with compassion and journal how that helped you.

SUNDAY

If you have already completed the previous six days this week, then this is a free day to spend an hour doing something that you really love to do, that supports your recovery. If you're not where you want to be in this work, do it today.

Meditate.

https://www.youtube.com/watch?v=AGXHWm7rVoQ&ab_channel=CarrieSchell

Give yourself time today to be still for a few moments to give thanks for the journey you are on. This is not easy. A lot is coming up, a lot is changing.

Know in your heart and mind that it is all for the good.

Week 4

Okay, so now you're noticing mind, body, spirit benefits of doing the reset.

Hopefully your body has begun to feel different because of the physical activity, mindfulness, and healthy eating.

You'll also notice that your thoughts and way of being in the world is starting to shift. At first the changes may be subtle and barely noticeable. Then one day, you'll simply become aware that you are not doing things the same way anymore.

If you haven't noticed too many changes, maybe you haven't been sticking with the program each day and that's okay. Be kind to yourself and don't stress about it.

If this is you, what do you do? Do you quit? Definitely not! Maybe you want to recommit and start the program from where you left off. Maybe you're the kind of person who wants to go back to week one and start over. The choice is yours.

But it's my true hope that you will just do it. Just keep this book open and read. Go for a walk or whatever you enjoy doing and connect with your body. Listen to the meditation and simply be. Honour yourself. Love yourself.

I recommend that you take some time and meditate on what you do next and where you can reimmerse yourself in the program. It will become clear to you. The cool thing is that you can start again anytime you want. With this book as your guide, you can do this on your terms. By taking a moment to reflect, your next steps will become more clear to you.

All I can tell you is that if you can just stay with it, you will reconnect with your mind, body, and spirit. This is your journey. It is my intention to support you in your work.

We all make commitments we find difficult to live up to from time to time, but if we know they are commitments that are in our best interests, or ones we truly want to keep, then we recommit. We start over and do what we originally intended to do.

Just remember our goal when we started, to commit to one day at a time and it will all fall into place. You are worth it. Even if you have worked the program, you may want to go back from time to time and revisit certain sections that you find encouraging and supportive, the ones that truly spoke to you. Each time you do, you'll get something new out of it.

Believe it or not, you are blessed to be in a place where you have the choice to be doing this mind, body, spirit reset. What a gift to be present enough and well enough to engage in this challenge. *And that is why the theme for this week is choice.*

You know better than most that being able to be in a place where you can actually have choices takes time. It starts with when you begin to become aware, aware of where you are on your journey.

Once you develop an awareness, it is so important to be able to accept your awareness and to accept where you are. When we can see where we are, we are then able to also see the choices that lay before us.

Choices are available in every moment and in all we do – our thoughts, our actions, and even our emotions. Part of the beauty of clean living is having the clarity to of being in the moment, of being aware of our life as we are living it.

This "being in the moment" provides us with the opportunity to actively change our reality. We can choose our present moments. If our choices are not supporting us in creating what we want in our lives, then maybe we need to look at the choices we are making. Maybe we're making choices out of habit, or choices because they're expedient – a choice for a few fleeting moments of pleasure, the promise of better things to come, but at the end, not for real happiness.

At the start of this program, and each day when you set your intention, you are making a statement to yourself about what you are really seeking in life. As you become more aware of your intention and goals, you can continue to do what you've done in the past, or based on your new awareness, you can choose to do something different. You can choose something that will support a healthy life – mind, body, and spirit. It may not always be the easy choice, but when choices are made to support your intention of being present and healthy, they are always worth the effort, I promise.

Choice is powerful. It means we can move in new directions and bring about real change. Move slowly and carefully and begin with this one new change in your life. Take the time to feel the impact of this new choice and all of the benefits you are experiencing.

What will be helpful in making the smaller, day to day choices, is becoming aware of the choices you are currently making. Part of your practice this week will be to discover your choices by being more aware as you actively engage in each moment of the day.

Remember, you are moving from a place of no choice to a place of infinite potential. In doing so, we become the victor, not the victim. How great is that? And guess what? The power to choose to be victorious is all yours.

You have the power within you.

MONDAY

Two Minutes

Notice and Accepting ~ Focus and Intention Setting

Five Minutes

- Take at least five 20-second awareness breaks today.

- Practice accepting all that you notice.

- Notice what you are currently choosing.

- Meditation and Integration. The light in me honours the light in you.

https://www.youtube.com/watch?v=-LRvhHD82nI&t=7s&ab_channel=CarrieSchell

Thirty Minutes

- Physical activity.

- Drink 8 glasses of water today.

- Perform one small act to support your intention.

- Schedule a treat for your body later this week.

Today's Thought

Affirming your choices.

You are standing in the corridor of Life, and behind you so many doors have closed. Things you no longer do or say or think. Experiences you no longer have. Ahead of you is an unending corridor of doors ~ each one opening to a new experience.

As you move forward, see yourself opening various doors to wonderful experiences that you would like to have. Trust that your inner guide is leading you and guiding you in ways that are best for you, and that your spiritual growth is continuously expanding.

No matter which door opens or which door closes, you are always safe. You are eternal. You will go on forever from experience to experience. See yourself opening doors to joy, peace, healing, prosperity, and love. Doors to understanding, compassion, and forgiveness. Doors to self-love. It is all here before you. Which door will you open first?

Remember you are safe. This is only healing change.

Word for the Day: *CHANGE*

"The key to change...is to let go of fear."

~Rosanne Cash

"All changes, even the most longed for, have their melancholy; for what we leave behind us is a part of ourselves; we must die to one life before we can enter another."

~Anatole France

"Any change, even a change for the better,

is always accompanied by drawbacks ad discomforts."

~Arnold Bennett

Isn't it absolutely baffling how we can want change, we can know that change will only serve us, and we can even know that change is inevitable and yet we resist! I mean, take drinking. I knew I was drinking too much. I knew that it was becoming an issue, that I was longing for a glass of wine each day. I knew that my husband and I were creating unhealthy drinking patterns as a couple. And I knew that I wanted to be stronger, healthier, an amazing role model to my kids, showing them that yeah, I loved my glass of wine, but I love them, and I love me way, way more than wine.

And so, we embrace change while at the same time we resist change. But whatever you are thinking or feeling in this moment, know that because you had the awareness of the need to explore grey drinking and to *change*, the change has happened. It may not have fully matured, it may still be in its infancy, but the fact that you are aware you need to change means it is inevitable.

It is coming. It may take weeks and months to be so friggin' happy you made the change, but change you will. You've already begun.

Affirmation

I now seek to find joy in all things life has given me.

Journaling

This week we are going to express the various choices we have made that brought us to today. They can be choices that had negative consequences, or they can be choices that had a positive impact on our lives.

It is important to start showing up in the decision-making process and taking ownership for our actions. Becoming aware of the choices we have made and why we made them is key to this.

Understanding how we have chosen in the past will help direct the choices we make in the future with intention, positive intention. This is not meant to be a self-flagellating exercise. We have all experienced the good, the bad, and the ugly. The intention is to bring understanding, awareness, and the appreciation that we govern our choices.

Excerpt

Sometimes when I am alone and driving, listening to music, I can get this feeling of deep sadness. Not often, just sometimes. I'm not sad about anything in particular. Nothing has happened to bring on the feeling. It simply appears. It is subtle, not overwhelming, just there.

And I think to myself, "Why am I feeling this way? Things are good. I am good. I have a loving husband and great family. I've been blessed with my work life, and I have a deep spiritual life."

And then I think of how I have a really shitty memory. I just have vague memories of my childhood, more feelings surrounding certain periods than clear memories. And I think of how incredible the brain is to grant us this ability of not remembering. I didn't have a traumatic childhood but there is a sadness rooted there.

I also think that I am so blessed that for most of my life I was never upset or angry when my parents got divorced and with all the dysfunction that followed. It wasn't until I was having Christian (my son) that I began to remember how my parents could behave, and how they did towards us. Is that when I started drinking more regularly?

Exercise

Describe what changes you need to make at this point in your journey in order to live sober and happy in this moment, on this day.

TUESDAY

Two Minutes

Notice and Accepting ~ Focus and Intention Setting

Five Minutes

- Take at least five 20-second awareness breaks today.

- Practice accepting all that you notice.

- Notice what you are currently choosing.

- Meditation and Integration. Inhale…exhale…

https://www.youtube.com/watch?v=S03R-Gxrszg&t=328s&ab_channel=CarrieSchell

Thirty Minutes

- Physical activity.

- Drink 8 glasses of water today.

- Perform one small act to support your intention.

- Schedule a treat for your body later this week.

Today's Thought

Do whatever it takes.

In the beginning, and for as long as it takes, do whatever you have to do to keep yourself from drinking. It may mean clear out all alcohol from your home, no dinner parties, brunches and girl's lunches, but do whatever it takes.

I know this sounds super drastic but cravings will surface and when they do, you do not want to give into the temptation due to easy access.

When that craving surfaces, take whatever action is called for. Phone a friend who can come to your side. Or get out of yourself and think of others, call someone you know who has been having a difficult time and ask how you can help. Turn the tables. Help yourself by helping another. You might listen to music, read a book. Take a bath. Visit somebody. Go see a movie. Go to a bookstore. Do yoga. Meditate. Pray. Play.

These are simple suggestions. You will find others to help you ride out the craving. When you don't give into it, a craving is a sort-lived entity, even powerful ones that seem to overwhelm you, and make you rationalize to yourself all the reasons you should have that glass of wine get easier.

Find the strength to resist. Remember how good you felt when you first became aware you were okay not drinking and feeling healthy. Remember how in those moments you never wanted to go back to drinking. These craving will eventually stop when they aren't fed. Ride them out often enough and they will get the message that there is no use in bothering you any longer.

Word for Today: *LOVE*

"Take away love and our earth is a tomb."

~Robert Browning

"The kind of love that the greatest thinkers and saviours of the world talked about is very different from what most people understand love to be. It is much more than loving your family, friends, and favourite things, because love is not just a feeling: love is a positive force. Love is not weak, feeble, or soft. Love is the positive force of life. Love is the cause of everything positive and good. There are not a hundred different positive forces in life: there is only one."

~Rhonda Bryne, *The Power*

Love is a state of consciousness. In order to truly experience love, that unyielding, never-ending love we all need and long for, you must release all that is not love from within you.

On this journey we are learning to notice, become aware, have compassion, and now we need to learn to love in a way that is healthy and supports us. We need to learn to love without expectations or wants, but simply to give to those around us.

When you have love in your heart there is no room for hate, cruelty, judgements, and criticisms. Love sees beauty where others see ugliness. Love honours nature and appreciates each day of life as a new opportunity to express love. Love is full of laughter, joy, and wisdom. Love is the highest and best expression in us all.

Affirmation

Love is the cause of everything positive and good.

Journaling

This week we are going to express the various choices we have made that brought us to today. They can be choices that had negative consequences or they can be choices that had a positive impact on our lives.

It is important to start showing up in the decision-making process and taking ownership for our actions. Becoming aware of the choices we have made and why we made them is key to this.

Understanding how we have chosen in the past will help direct the choices we make in the future with intention, positive intention. This is not meant to be a self-flagellating exercise. We have all experienced the good, the bad, and the ugly. The intention is to bring understanding, awareness, and the appreciation that we govern our choices.

Excerpt

I am feeling a quiet calm. I am waking up having slept better, deeper. I'm not congested. Can alcohol make you congested? I'll have to look that one up.

Although I was never one to think about having a drink during the day or planning when I would have that first glass of wine, something is different. Something is changing and it's a good change. I can just feel it.

Nothing has changed since I went to bed last night, but it is almost as though I am stepping into something new. I'm on the precipice and I am fully leading the way. Even though before I was a determined, hard-working person, it always literally tormented me that I could not get this drinking thing to a place I felt

good about. There was always this secret co-pilot navigating a certain course in my life.

But today feels different. Today feels new. Today feels good.

Exercise

Write of love – your memories and experiences of what love feels like.

Please keep this exercise only positive. Remember the goodness and happiness of love, wherever it has existed in your life.

WEDNESDAY

Two Minutes

Notice and Accepting ~ Focus and Intention Setting

Five Minutes

- Take at least five 20-second awareness breaks today.

- Practice accepting all that you notice.

- Notice what you are currently choosing.

- Meditation and Integration. Inhale…exhale…

https://www.youtube.com/watch?v=OTzP3a_50T4&t=10s&ab_channel=CarrieSchell

Thirty Minutes

- Physical activity.

- Drink 8 glasses of water today.

- Perform one small act to support your intention.

- Schedule a treat for your body later this week.

Today's Thought

Be present in today.

Today is the day you've got. Do not set overwhelming goals for yourself. The tiny changes you are making each day will add up. Just stay in today.

When you live for today, you stay in the present, living out the work of not drinking. Today is it, and what you do today is all that matters.

Staying centered in the now keeps you aware of what you're doing. You will be far less likely to give into defeatist thoughts and behaviors. When you stay focused, you experience the day ~ its events, its sensations, its nuances. Life will become richer and more gratifying. You will have fewer regrets because regrets belong to the past. You will worry less because worry is about the future, and when the future becomes the present, it won't be nearly as frightening ~ the present almost never is.

Keeping your focus on the here and now also makes it possible to live the way you want to. An incentive for staying in today is that this is where everything is happening: life, pleasure, accomplishment, and most importantly LOVE.

Today is where it all happens, and you are already here. Live it. Love it.

Word for Today: *FORGIVENESS*

"Forgiveness is giving up the idea of having a better past. 'I can forgive, but I cannot forget' is only another way of saying, 'I will not forgive.' Forgiveness ought to be like a cancelled note – torn in two, and burned up, so that it can never be shown against one."

~Henry Ward Beecher

"The weak can never forgive. Forgiveness is the attribute of the strong."
~Mahatma Gandhi

There are three essential parts to self-forgiveness:

1. Acknowledge having acted in the wrong and accept responsibility for that wrong.

2. Allow yourself to experience feelings of guilt and regret.

3. Overcome these feelings through forgiveness and self-forgiveness and in doing so, experience a motivational change away from self-punishment toward self-acceptance.

Forgiveness for me is a battle between good and evil, between the positive and the negative, between the present and the past, between being in flow or not.

When our hearts and minds are focused on the power of goodness, we are unstoppable. The impossible becomes possible. Here's what I do know: we are vulnerably human. Even though we extend forgiveness to ourselves and others, we will inevitably have moments when those negative emotions resurface.

And here's another thing I know. For me, most of my challenges with forgiveness come from feeling less than worthy. I lose sight that I am a beautiful divine spirit that doesn't need another's praise or approval to be of value. I am of infinite worth simply because I am here.

When I forget that, that's when shit hits the fan. I live in the past, rehashing old wounds, stirring negative emotions. When you feel you are being pulled out of flow, take a moment or two and ground yourself. Remember that the Divine dwells within you. You are worthy.

When you focus on this, forgiveness becomes easy, a joy, a gift to extend.

Affirmation

Forgiveness of myself and others sets me free from the past.

Journaling

This week we are going to express the various choices we have made that have brought us to today. They can be choices that had negative consequences or they can be choices that had a positive impact on our lives.

It is important to start showing up in the decision-making process and taking ownership for our actions. Becoming aware of the choices we have made and why we made them is key to this.

Understanding how we have chosen in the past will help direct the choices we make in the future with intention, positive intention. This is not meant to be a self-flagellating exercise. We have all experienced the good, the bad, and the ugly. The intention is to bring understanding, awareness, and the appreciation that we govern our choices.

Excerpt

How are people going to react to me not drinking? It's not that I was ever this crazy, party girl drunk, it's just that I know friends and family are going to look at me different. Almost like, "Sure, let's see how long this lasts."

I also think that when someone who enjoyed having drinks doesn't anymore, through no action of their own, it turns the mirror glass onto those around them, making them take a look at themselves and their own drinking behaviours.

At this point, I don't give a shit. I need to do this for me. Change is a-comin' and everyone better get used to it.

Exercise

What experience lays heavy on your heart? Do you need to forgive yourself or someone else to restore peace within you? What stands in your way? Is it pride, anger, righteousness, or stubbornness?

Be honest with yourself as you begin to explore the miraculous power of forgiveness.

THURSDAY

Two Minutes

Notice and Accepting ~ Focus and Intention Setting

Five Minutes

- Take at least five 20-second awareness breaks today.

- Practice accepting all that you notice.

- Notice what you are currently choosing.

- Meditation and Integration. Inhale…exhale…

https://www.youtube.com/watch?v=deH14yUg5Q4&ab_channel=CarrieSchell

Thirty Minutes

- Physical activity.

- Drink 8 glasses of water today.

- Perform one small act to support your intention.

- Schedule a treat for your body later this week.

Today's Thought

Never punish yourself.

There are all sorts of ways to punish yourself for your situation. A negative, punishing attitude toward yourself won't help you in your goal to live a healthy life not dependent on alcohol.

Instead, know that when you're setting positive intentions it is always good enough! If you have fallen short, now is the time to begin again. Treat yourself with the love and kindness you would offer someone else who is struggling and allow yourself the space to move forward.

Getting through the dependence on alcohol can be challenging enough without you being your own worst enemy. Love starts here, from within. Let the flicker of self-love grow from within until it radiates outward. Simply allow yourself the room you need to grow and step into your fullness.

If you have been punitive and defeatist in the past, watch what you say to yourself, both inside and outside your head. Watch for the subtle ways you punish yourself. Don't see yourself in terms of failure. Keep yourself in the safety of this day. This will help make setbacks less likely. When you disappoint yourself, treat yourself the way you would treat your best friend or child in a similar circumstance.

Be a friend to yourself. Learn the lessons life presents. And in the meantime, let yourself grow, heal, renew, rejuvenate, and triumph.

Word for Today: *RESPECT*

"To be respectful is an attitude of caring about the feelings of others. To have self-respect means that you have become aware of how precious life is and live your life reflecting this. A caring attitude towards oneself, others, and the earth demonstrates someone rooted in love, gratitude, and grace. If you want to be respected by others, the great thing is to respect yourself. Only by that, only by self-respect will you compel others to respect you."

~Fyodor Dostoyevsky

I think today the word respect is often associated with power, status, wealth and influence. When we look at the definition of respect we see that really, respect is a reflection of one's true character and emotions.

Respect

"A feeling of deep admiration for someone or something…" "Due regard for the feelings, wishes and rights, or traditions of others."

Shifting the essence of respect from the external to the internal is important for our work together. Your initial questioning of your drinking habits propelled you into action to begin the 30 day reset. It is my hope that your dedication and determination to regain control in your relationship with alcohol will cultivate within you a feeling of deep admiration for you! You began this journey because you listened to that voice within, and gave due regard to your true feelings, wishes and *rights* to be free from the stronghold of alcohol. You have honoured yourself with **respect.**

Affirmation

I now cultivate an understanding that all deserve respect, myself included.

Journaling

This week we are going to express the various choices we have made that have brought us to today. They can be choices that had negative consequences, or they can be choices that had a positive impact on our lives.

It is important to start showing up in the decision-making process and taking ownership for our actions. Becoming aware of the choices we have made and why we made them is key to this.

Understanding how we have chosen in the past will help direct the choices we make in the future with intention, positive intention. This is not meant to be a self-flagellating exercise. We have all experienced the good, the bad, and the ugly. The intention is to bring understanding, awareness, and the appreciation that we govern our choices.

Excerpt

What is the line between being a good "host" and being a pusher? Am I a pusher rather than a gracious hostess? When we all get together, I know I am always quick to offer the kids a drink but that isn't because I want to get drunk or get them drunk. I am trying to be warm and inviting and let them enjoy a family evening.

But is it too much? Do I have to rethink all of that? What is the balance there? Thankfully the kids aren't big drinkers. Shit, is that because of us? They are so much smarter than we are. They are amazing humans who I love deeply. I need to find that balance between being gracious and pushy.

Exercise

Remember a time you were treated with disrespect. Write what the word respect means to you and how you are cultivating this attitude within you.

FRIDAY

Two Minutes

Notice and Accepting ~ Focus and Intention Setting

Five Minutes

- Take at least five 20-second awareness breaks today.

- Practice accepting all that you notice.

- Notice what you are currently choosing.

- Meditation and Integration. Let it all go with a guided meditation.

https://www.youtube.com/watch?v=FpLp7waxoNU&ab_channel=CarrieSchell

Thirty Minutes

- Physical activity.

- Drink 8 glasses of water today.

- Perform one small act to support your intention.

- Schedule a treat for your body later this week.

Today's Thought

Tap into your courage.

Courage is not just about people who save lives or make headlines. We all have courage. We have the potential to live with courage in our everyday lives.

The courage you need for most days is subtle. It's the courage that allows you to abstain from drinking. It's the courage that allows you to be present in your life, your family, your marriage, your work. It's the courage to smile when you're struggling the most.

Courage is an odd quality in that you may have a great deal of it in one area and virtually none in another. You may have no idea how brave you are until you are facing your first challenge or trigger.

On this journey, the greatest courage you can demonstrate is the ability to say no, walk away, and not drink. It takes courage to put yourself out there, trust in others, and develop new relationships that are healthy and supportive. It can create fears, for sure. Reduce fear by taking each day as it comes. Deal with various stressors (relationships, overscheduling, finances) and be so good to yourself on the ordinary days that you'll be up to the challenge of difficult days.

Whether you feel you need more courage to deal with not drinking or with other issues, calling upon your higher power will strengthen your resolve. When you're counting on your higher power or a higher purpose, you've got a light to help you through the dark places.

Word for the Day: *TOLERANCE*

"Surely the day will come when colour means nothing more than skin tone, when religion is seen uniquely as a way to speak one's soul; when birth places have the weight of a throw of a dice and all men are born free, when understanding breeds love and brotherhood."

~Josephine Baker

"It is thus tolerance that is the source of peace, and intolerance that is the source of disorder and squabbling."

~Peter Bayle

In the context of the work that we are doing together, tolerance, for me, takes on a different meaning. Here we are, Friday of week four. We're feeling good, strong, amazed that we have made it this far without drinking. Not even that, it is getting *easier.* Okay, maybe not always easier, but more manageable and realistic.

This journey has most definitely opened your eyes to patterns of behaviour of those around you, a partner, friends, co-workers, parents. So, what do we do when we recognize unhealthy drinking in *them?* What do we do when the people we relied on, socialized with, are now presenting us with potential stumbling blocks to our success?

We exercise tolerance. Not a lip-biting tolerance, but a tolerance that extends genuine love and understanding to where others are at on their journey. We have an incredible opportunity to share with others, simply by example, that we can live a fuller, healthier, happier, more present life without the blinders of alcohol.

We love them. And in doing so, we are truly tolerant.

Affirmation

I now seek to practice tolerance by understanding myself and others.

Journaling

This week we are going to express the various choices we have made that brought us to today. They can be choices that had negative consequences, or they can be choices that had a positive impact on our lives.

It is important to start showing up in the decision-making process and taking ownership for our actions. Becoming aware of the choices we have made and why we made them is key to this.

Understanding how we have chosen in the past will help direct the choices we make in the future with intention, positive intention. This is not meant to be a self-flagellating exercise. We have all experienced the good, the bad, and the ugly. The intention is to bring understanding, awareness, and the appreciation that we govern our choices.

Excerpt

I really do believe mothers carry a lot of guilt. I carry a lot of guilt. Everything just always seems to be my fault. It just seems as if there are any failures, disappointments, fears, it can all come back to me.

And I can't really disagree. Divorce is shitty, no matter how you look at it, no matter if it was for the "best." When marriages go through really bad times and impact the kids...I can own it all. I no longer blame myself, but I can't ignore that. I understand and appreciate the negative impact it has had on the kids and for that I could never have another glass of wine from here until eternity and it would never erase that impact, would never be enough.

Exercise

"In the practice of tolerance, one's enemy is the best teacher."

~14th Dalai Lama

Think of a person that has helped you learn the lesson of tolerance. What was the lesson? How did this help you grow?

SATURDAY

Two Minutes

Notice and Accepting ~ Focus and Intention Setting

Five Minutes

- Take at least five 20-second awareness breaks today.

- Practice accepting all that you notice.

- Notice what you are currently choosing.

- Meditation and Integration. Simply breathe with a guided meditation.
https://www.youtube.com/watch?v=-HhSnob0DUw&ab_channel=CarrieSchell

Thirty Minutes

- Physical activity.

- Drink 8 glasses of water today.

- Perform one small act to support your intention.

- Schedule a treat for your body later this week.

- Smile and do yoga.

Today's Thought

Stop comparing.

Stop comparing yourself to friends, strangers, and earlier versions of yourself. Comparing is a game that nobody wins. We are all worthy. Our being alive, being present in this world, gives us an inherent worthiness that can never be diminished or taken from us.

Comparing is a vicious cycle because it always means we are viewing someone or something as lesser – and usually it's hard not feel we are the lesser. Let's make every effort to move away from that pattern of thought. It can never be a positive, growing experience. There is enough abundance in the universe – no one has to be the lesser.

Support your friends who are trying to succeed and grow and know that you deserve the same unconditional backing, whether others know how to give it to you or not. And when anyone you know has a triumph in any area of life, celebrate with them. Be part of the exhilaration of somebody else's accomplishments. Blessings are contagious: be there for them and they will, in return, be there for you.

We have this mistaken belief that there are limits in life – limits to joy, happiness, love, abundance, and prosperity, to whatever. These limiting beliefs make us feel that when someone else experiences success in some area of their life, it somehow diminishes or takes away from the potential for us to experience that same triumph.

There is a limitless supply in the universe, and there are no limits on what you seek. Set your intentions and put it out there. The more we celebrate the victories and triumphs of others, the more we will receive.

Whatever you feel about yourself today, and whether or not you believe you deserve it, make a commitment to take loving care of yourself as you are right now. Savour the time you spend with the people that matter and on the parts of your life that bring you the most happiness.

There's no need to compare yourself to anybody else because you are one of a kind. Other people have every right to be beautiful, prosperous, powerful, madly in love, or mildly in ecstasy. The absolutely amazing this is, so do you!

Word for Today: *JOY*

"Worry never robs tomorrow of its sorrow, it only saps today of its joy."

~Leo Buscaglia

"Don't postpone joy until you have learned all of your lessons. Joy is your lesson."

~Alan Cohen

Joy is an essential spiritual practice growing out of faith, grace, gratitude, hope, and love. It's the pure and simple delight in being alive. Joy is our elated response to feelings of happiness, experiences of meaning, and awareness of abundance.

It's also the deep satisfaction when we are able to serve others and delight in someone else's good fortune. Joy is being able to feel peace while experiencing challenges. Joy is beyond good times felt in the moment. Joy is a deep, sustained relationship with our higher self, our true self.

Joy is knowing you without alcohol.

Affirmation

I now seek to find joy in all things life has given me.

Journaling

This week we are going to express the various choices we have made that brought us to today. They can be choices that had negative consequences or they can be choices that had a positive impact on our lives.

It is important to start showing up in the decision-making process and taking ownership for our actions. Becoming aware of the choices we have made and why we made them is key to this.

Understanding how we have chosen in the past will help direct the choices we make in the future with intention, positive intention. This is not meant to be a self-flagellating exercise. We have all experienced the good, the bad, and the ugly. The intention is to bring understanding, awareness, and the appreciation that we govern our choices.

Excerpt

I have such a sense of relief. I think that would be the overarching emotion I am experiencing right now.

I am relieved that after so many years of wondering if I drink too much, wondering if I should cut back, wondering if I should stop at all, that I have finally found the time and space to do it. I am a grey drinker. ***I am a grey drinker*** *and that is okay.*

I feel the relief of when you have an illness and have no clue what is causing it and the doctor finally gives you a diagnosis and you get this sense of peace in knowing that at least now you know what you're up against. I know what I'm up against. I drink too much. I have enjoyed drinking too much and it is time to let it go.

I don't know if grey drinkers can ever drink again. I don't know if I want to be the one to experiment with the notion. I know that I am feeling alert, bright, happy, proud, content, and relieved. I know that the grace of God has helped me and is helping me to step into all I am meant to be and that doesn't include a woman who needs alcohol. I am thankful. I am blessed. I am honoured and grateful to be on this journey. Maybe my story will help other "grey women." Maybe. But for today I am simply being me and it is always more than enough.

Exercise

Explore how joy can be found even in face of adversity. Was there ever a time when you experienced a moment of joy even in the midst of heartache?

SUNDAY

It's week four, you know the drill.

Take the time today to go back to a day you may have missed or do something else you love to do or maybe go crazy and try something you've always longed to do.

Just be kind to you. You are so lovely and wonderful.

Enjoy the peace a guided meditation brings.

https://www.youtube.com/watch?v=AGXHWm7rVoQ&ab_channel=CarrieSchell

Day 30

Wow! We are done! Can you believe it? Where did those 30 days go?

Today is a time for reflection. You've done the heavy lifting and now I want you to take some time to do an honest assessment of how this journey has been for you.

My intention is that you will have clarity of thought with respect to your relationship with alcohol. If this has been incredibly difficult for you, a struggle every step of the way, hopefully this will signal that your relationship with alcohol is not healthy and that you need to either continue this program or find another way to develop behaviours to support you and a healthy approach to drinking.

If you are finding that you loved the changes you have been experiencing, I want you to take time to let that truly sink in. Do you want to continue on this path of positivity, growth, and creating opportunities for a healthier you? I encourage you not to be so quick to go back to alcohol. It can be very tempting, now that the 30 days are over, to celebrate your success with a drink or two. I hope that reading this it strikes you as how counter intuitive that is. Celebrating feeling incredible for not drinking for 30 days by drinking, crazy! But we are crazy creatures and that is precisely the kind of thing we do. We diet, lose weight, and *then* eat the cake.

Now is a time for prayer, meditation, and reflection. What are your next steps? You are in control. You, and only you, determine what your next steps will be.

Take the Bliss Test again and compare it your first one. Have your responses shifted? My hope for you is that you have experienced positive changes somewhere along the journey.

Making life changes takes time. You may have struggled more than you anticipated, and that's okay! Anything truly worthwhile takes determination, effort, willpower, and faith.

I am here for you. We can continue this journey together. You aren't alone.

Today, celebrate the wonderful being that is you! You had the insight and courage to acknowledge that the ways you were being didn't support the best version of you.

Thank you! Thank you for letting me be with you for these past 30 days. Thank you for being you. It is always, always enough.

Sending light and love!

Carrie

Simple Bliss Test

Now that you have completed the Reset, retake the Bliss Test and see how you have changed. You may be surprised.

This test is not meant to be used as a scientific tool, but a fun way to give you an overall idea of the extent of stress and bliss in your life.

Rate each item on a scale of 0 to 10 in terms of how accurately it describes you.

A 0 would be "Does not describe me at all."

A 5 would be "Sometimes describes me."

A 10 would be "Always describes me."

1. I am a happy person.

2. I have a clear purpose in my life that I'm pleased about.

3. I am achieving what I want in my life.

4. The stress in my life is moderate to manageable.

5. I am patient and calm in times of struggle.

6. I take good care of my physical and emotional health.

7. My life is exciting and challenging.

8. I get pleasure regularly from helping others.

9. There are people in my life who love me and who I enjoy spending time with.

10. My work is meaningful to me and serves others.

Total score out of a possible 100 ____

Results

If you scored 0-30, you don't have a lot of bliss in your life, and you're probably experiencing one or more symptoms of stress.

If you scored 31-60, you could probably use more bliss in your life, but you may not notice you feel all that stressed out.

If you scored 61-100, spread the love.

New Beginnings

Wow. Four weeks have passed. Thank you for including me. I am truly honoured. Now it's time to take a moment to reflect on your journey.

If you have followed the program perfectly for the four weeks, that's incredible. You will undoubtedly feel stronger, healthier, and more empowered. If you have struggled to stay with the program and have done only bits and pieces, that's okay. Hopefully that will be enough for you to know that it's worth the effort, and more importantly, that you are worth the time and effort.

We all struggle. There is no pass or fail. Please do not stress and simply allow yourself the freedom to make a clean start and try the program again from the beginning.

As you look back and notice how much or little of the program you were able to stay with, celebrate all you have learned. What stood out as an important turning point and how has that affected your life? Are you any clearer in the understanding that you direct your life and have the power to turn your stress into bliss? This is a huge learning and in time you will come to know that it is a blessing.

My hope is that you have been able to make a difference in your life over the past four weeks. So, where do you go now? What do you want to build into your life that will continue to support you in creating the reality you want?

If you want to create more bliss and less stress in your life in the future, you need to set up your life in ways that will support this intention. What aspects of this mind, body, spirit reset have created the space to be able to bring more joy into your life?

It is not easy to live your life mindfully. It is much easier to just react to situations as they come up. It's easier to be the victim of circumstance than it is to choose the path that will make a positive difference. Taking time daily to care for yourself gives you breathing space to allow you to remember what it is you really want and need to do in order to continue in that desired direction. This way of being takes awareness, patience, compassion, understanding, love, and courage.

Some people believe that courage means facing ordeals without fear or resistance, like the warrior going into battle. In truth, the real hero, the real warrior, is not the one without fear and resistance, but the one who feels fear and resistance, acknowledges it, and goes for it anyway. Even when we are committed to change our lives and live more fully, we will still experience resistance and fear somewhere along the way. That's normal, and that is okay.

Knowing what to do when you encounter resistance and fear is going to serve you on your wellness journey and beyond. If you acknowledge your triggers and stressors and are committed to the new path you are presently on, you will be able to dig deep and access the skills you have practiced in the last four weeks.

Developing a life of wellness means committing to your life's journey, in its entirety, including a spiritual practice. Our physical and spiritual meditation practice reminds us that there is no quick fix. It's about developing a deep and meaningful relationship with oneself and others through the trials and joys of life. This is why in yoga and the setting of our intention is so vital. The intention of our meditation practice is to become a more peaceful, happy, and joyful person.

But here's the thing: we live in a society that believes that it is possible to live in a pain-free, quick solution, immediate satisfaction environment. Unfortunately, we are rarely taught how to develop the tools to deal with the realities of life, with all the struggles and challenges. We aren't taught to value the growth that comes with challenges, and to appreciate and welcome how it is through our hardships that we are able to become the best versions of ourselves.

Wellness and recovery are not about getting rid of all the challenges we face or by ignoring them or controlling our environment. It's about keeping our peace of mind and sense of self regardless of whether you experience ease and flow or stuckness and difficulties.

This is why it's crucial that you get the clarity you need, and the resolve needed to confront your triggers and stressors before they take you somewhere you don't want to be. You must understand the true value of happiness as opposed to feeling good in the moment. Remember, to develop this understanding you need to cultivate an awareness of where you are in the moment. It's this understanding that gives us the power to choose our next steps. It is my hope and intention that our work together will support your intentions of being present and living a life of wellness.

It's a very different approach to life than what many of us know or have been taught to follow. This is an ongoing journey to deeper levels of knowledge of awareness and happiness. It is a journey that requires courage, commitment, self-generated power, and above all, the recognition within us that we are unique and wonderful human beings. It is the journey of self-worthiness. It is the journey to you, without barriers or distractions, to the Spirit within you, your true Self, your Divine self.

You are worthy. You have made it here with a purpose. It is no accident that you have decided to take this journey with me, to be reading this, seriously.

You are a miracle. Never forget that. There is light within you.

God bless you and Namaste,

Carrie

A Final Note from Carrie

Wow.

I suppose the most important thing to know about me is that this book comes from a source of love with the intention of being in service to you.

I feel blessed to have created this work and am overwhelmed with gratitude for your allowing me to be with you on this journey.

God bless and Namaste.

"And in the end the love you take is equal to the love you make."

~The Beatles

CPSIA information can be obtained
at www.ICGtesting.com
Printed in the USA
BVHW090756101222
653840BV00005B/253